NEW DIRECTIONS FOR MENTAL HEALTH SERVICES

H. Richard Lamb, *University of Southern California*
EDITOR-IN-CHIEF

Using Psychodynamic Principles in Public Mental Health

Terry A. Kupers
The Wright Institute

EDITOR

Number 46, Summer 1990

JOSSEY-BASS INC., PUBLISHERS
San Francisco • Oxford

Using Psychodynamic Principles in Public Mental Health.
Terry A. Kupers (ed.).
New Directions for Mental Health Services, no. 46.

NEW DIRECTIONS FOR MENTAL HEALTH SERVICES
H. Richard Lamb, Editor-in-Chief

Microfilm copies of issues and articles are available in 16mm and
35mm, as well as microfiche in 105mm, through University Microfilms
Inc., 300 North Zeeb Road, Ann Arbor, Michigan 48106.

NEW DIRECTIONS FOR MENTAL HEALTH SERVICES is part of The Jossey-
Bass Social and Behavioral Sciences Series and is published quarterly
by Jossey-Bass Inc., Publishers (publication number USPS 493-910).
Second-class postage paid at San Francisco, California, and at
additional mailing offices. Postmaster: Send address changes to
Jossey-Bass Inc., Publishers, 350 Sansome Street, San Francisco,
California 94104.

EDITORIAL CORRESPONDENCE should be sent to the Editor-in-Chief,
H. Richard Lamb, Department of Psychiatry and the Behavioral
Sciences, U.S.C. School of Medicine, 1934 Hospital Place,
Los Angeles, California 90033.

Library of Congress Catalog Card Number LC 87-646993

International Standard Serial Number ISSN 0193-9416

International Standard Book Number ISBN 1-55542-833-9

Cover photograph by Wernher Krutein/PHOTOVAULT, copyright © 1990.
Manufactured in the United States of America. Printed on acid-free paper.

CONTENTS

Editor's Notes

Public Therapy: The Practice of Psychotherapy in the Public Mental Health Clinic (Kupers, 1981) began with a statement of the book's two aims: "One is to share with therapists some techniques, experiences, and ideas about how to adapt what they know of psychotherapy to the realities of practice in the public mental health clinic. The other is to introduce a wider readership to some of those realities: the plight of low-income clients; the repercussions of inadequate budgets on the quality of public mental health services; the substitution of external controls where psychotherapy is not possible; and the conflicts and problems the therapist faces when attempting to practice in such a setting" (p. 1). These goals apply to this volume, as well, but recent changes in social context and in the structure of mental health services require therapists and other providers to make new adaptations of psychodynamic principles.

The last ten years have witnessed new social tragedies. Ones that are particularly relevant to mental health practitioners include the unprecedented use of crack cocaine and other drugs in urban areas along with the associated violence and social upheaval, plant closings, widespread homelessness, the spread of AIDS in the gay community as well as among needle users in the inner city, the worsening plight of the elderly, new outbreaks of racism and bigotry, and the traumatic effects of all of these developments on children. Changes in the social climate affect the condition of those already suffering from severe mental disorders, and they create new varieties of mental distress; consider, for example, the focus on homelessness and dual diagnosis in mental health circles today.

During the same ten years, shifts in social priorities have resulted in drastic cutbacks in social services, including the mental health delivery system. Of course, the consumers of mental health services are doubly affected: First, the safety net of employment opportunities, housing, and welfare benefits is much weaker, and then, when they find themselves in need of mental health services, there are fewer available. Fiscal accountability reigns in mental health departments. Limits to services are established. Such limits might mean briefer hospital stays or a shorter time limit for each client in a day-treatment or halfway house program; they might mean stricter limits on the number of psychotherapy sessions in an outpatient clinic or longer waits and less resources for vocational rehabilitation services; or they might mean that local mental health departments, when the time comes to finalize the next year's budget proposal, must select the least staff-intensive community program they can find—whether or not it is best for the clients and the community.

The idea behind deinstitutionalization was that when mental patients left the institutions, there would be resources available in the community to provide treatment programs and adequate housing and to prepare them to work and function as well as they could (Bachrach and Lamb, 1989). The reality fails to approximate the vision (Solomon, Davis, and Gordon, 1984). Cutbacks in social services cause many ex-hospital patients and many of the newer breed of never-hospitalized and dual-diagnosed young chronic patients (Pepper, Kirshner, and Ryglewicz, 1981; Brown and others, 1989) to join the ranks of the homeless and the unemployed. Their material circumstances do not make it any easier to treat their psychopathology.

Why is it important to talk about psychotherapy and psychodynamic principles today, when brief hospitalization, psychopharmacotherapy, case management, and community support programs seem so much the order of the day in public mental health? There are several reasons. Clinicians in many settings still consider the one-to-one therapeutic relationship an important component of community support programs for the seriously mentally disabled (Lamb, 1982, 1988). Then there are special populations in need of psychotherapy—the homeless, the elderly, those with a dual diagnosis, blue-collar workers, AIDS sufferers, children, and so on—and therapists who work with these populations need to adapt the principles of psychotherapy to the needs of their patients. Also, clinicians whose jobs do not call on them to function as therapists—for instance, the staff of a halfway house or a consultant hired to facilitate consumers' efforts to shape the mental health delivery system—can borrow from their experience as psychotherapists while working in different capacities. Finally, the design, implementation, and management of new mental health programs can be usefully informed by the designers' and providers' thorough familiarity with psychodynamic principles.

There is another reason for discussing the use of psychodynamic principles in the public mental health context: training. In the spring of 1989, I taught a course at the graduate school of psychology at New College (San Francisco) on the practice of psychotherapy in the public mental health clinic. The majority of contributors to this sourcebook made presentations. Several students asked why, when they were planning to become private practitioners, they were being introduced to the practice of therapy in the public mental health system. I responded that there is a real need for competent clinicians to work in the public sector, and I was hoping they might change their minds about practicing exclusively in the private sector. At least, as mental health professionals, they should know about the plight of the severely mentally disabled and the realities of the public sector (Cutler and Lefley, 1988). In addition, even if they eventually enter private practice, they will probably spend some of their required internship time in a public mental health program, and they should begin thinking about how to adapt their clinical training to that setting. In general, if discussion of psychodynamics and therapeutic technique does not occur in public mental health settings, then those clinicians who wish to practice dynamic psychotherapy will be forced to leave the public sector for private practice, and many other talented clinicians will never even consider working with the chronically mental ill. This would be a great loss to both sectors.

In Chapter One in this volume, Gale G. Bataille, an experienced clinician serving as an administrator of a large county mental health system, discusses some trends in mental health delivery systems, including priority services for seriously mentally ill adults and other target populations, the growing importance of consumer advocacy and participation, the advent of involuntary outpatient care for noncompliant patients, and the emphasis on social rehabilitation and community support programs. After presenting an overview of these developments, she suggests that there is still an important place for psychodynamic principles, but clinicians must learn to practice a new kind of "environmental therapy."

As soon as a large number of patients were discharged from psychiatric hospitals, it became apparent that a significant proportion would repeatedly return to the hospital, in effect establishing a "revolving-door" phenomenon (Solomon and Doll, 1979). Case management evolved as a possible solution. The idea is to assign the most difficult patients in a system (the ones with a high recidivism rate) to a few clinicians, then reduce those clinicians' caseloads and other responsibilities, and hope that their energetic case management will cut down the number of readmissions to the hospital (Harris and Bachrach, 1988). Cheryl M. Bryan, in Chapter Two, discusses the way a background in psychotherapy and a psychodynamic understanding can help the case manager carry out this rather large assignment.

Does psychotherapy benefit the chronic mental patient (Karon and Vandenbos, 1981; Glass and others, 1989), or is therapy only useful to the extent that the therapist is able to train the patient in the skills of daily living (Test and Stein, 1978)? In Chapter Three, Richard Bloom sidesteps a debate that has by now become polarized and shares some of his experience in working with the chronically mentally ill in an outpatient setting. Too often clinicians in this setting find it difficult to integrate what they read in the psychoanalytic literature with the mundane work they do from day to day. Bloom demonstrates how a contemporary psychoanalytic concept can be applied to the understanding of a severely disturbed man's antisocial behaviors. He also explores one way to understand the psychodynamics of chronicity. Meanwhile, he validates the feeling on the part of many clinicians who do this kind of work that in spite of pessimistic outcome studies, the work can improve the quality of patients' lives.

Necessity breeds invention. As federal, state, and local mental health departments place caps on budgets and lengths of treatment as well as mandate larger caseloads, the providers of public mental health services create innovative ways to supply effective services to a larger client population. The evolution of psychiatric or social rehabilitation programs (Anthony and Liberman, 1986), supported employment (Danley and Anthony, 1987), the use of continuous-treatment teams (Torrey, 1986), the training-in-community-living model (Stein and Test, 1985), as well as the concept of case management, are just a few examples. In halfway houses, day-treatment programs, assisted living programs, and community outreach services to the homeless, the elderly, or those suffering with AIDS, one finds dedicated mental health workers trying out new ways to serve the needs of their clientele. They gripe about the poor pay and the feeling that there are insufficient services available for their clients, but they try to do the best job they can within the constraints of limited budgets.

What is the place of psychotherapy or psychodynamic principles in community support programs? Many staff members in these programs are therapists or therapists in training, but their jobs do not specifically include doing therapy. Sometimes it is difficult to get therapists to do these other things. How does one get therapists to staff a halfway house without turning the work into one-on-one therapy? Once staff are able to settle into an appropriate role, however, a background in therapy is extremely useful in carrying out these other jobs. For instance, even in a vocational rehabilitation agency where therapy is not the main business at hand, when the staff member has some training in psychotherapeutics, he or she is better able to recognize a borderline client's pattern of acting out, to know when is the right time to offer insight and when the offer is likely to be refused, and to counter some of the client's failures by setting clear limits and confronting him or her firmly. Similarly, the halfway house counselor's background in psychotherapy is readily applied to the task of facilitating the venture in community living. Chapter Four describes how Elizabeth K. Gardner and the staff of the halfway house she directs have devised a creative way of analyzing the parallel process that occurs in a program designed to function as a therapeutic community.

How does one utilize psychodynamic principles in providing mental health services to the homeless? Christine A. Seeger, in Chapter Five, presents a psychosocial dynamic view of homelessness. She suggests that homelessness is a catastrophic event, a stressor equivalent to a war or a flood. Experience with the recent earthquake in the San Francisco Bay Area certainly demonstrates the acuity of the analogy. The first crisis needing attention was the grief of families who had lost members. Then there was an acute need for crisis intervention or "debriefing" among the exhausted rescue workers and emergency medical personnel. A week after the earthquake, the group who seemed most in need of assistance were those who had become homeless as a result of the disaster. Of course, the people with the least means were the ones needing the most ongoing assistance. The chronically mentally ill tend to fall into the last category—consider the plight of those housed in substandard inner-city transient hotels that crumbled or became uninhabitable after the earthquake. Seeger describes the process of becoming homeless as a downward spiral and suggests that providers who first understand and validate the homeless person's experience can then offer important services.

Mental patients are becoming advocates for and participants in a new generation of mental health programs. Ernest L. Silva's work (Chapter Six) is difficult to categorize. He is not exactly an advocate for clients and not really a provider of services, though he has played both roles in his work. Rather, he is someone who employs the therapist's sensibility to facilitate collaboration between providers and clients in the construction of a new kind of consumer-driven mental health program. Even though his focus is usually social dynamics rather than individual psychopathology, his insights and the interventions they inform have much in common with the practice of psychotherapy.

In Chapters One through Six, the volume focuses on the problems of the severely mentally disabled, a group that is targeted by Public Law 99-660. But there are other populations at risk and in need. Children, the elderly, and those who are dually diagnosed are targeted as well. And AIDS sufferers and blue-collar workers are populations that are too often ignored in discussions of community mental health. To borrow a term from traditional psychoanalysis, what "parameters" must we employ to reach these populations? In Chapter Seven, Lige Dailey, Jr., discusses his work with AIDS sufferers, offering not only some tips to the clinician on individual and family therapy but also his concern that so little attention is being paid to the inner-city AIDS epidemic. Here is a stark reminder of the double standard of mental health care delivery in our society—talking therapy for those who can afford private fees; for those less fortunate, minimal time to talk with caregivers. Does the sparseness of resources for the inner-city AIDS sufferer have anything to do with the fact that so many are minority members?

At a time when public mental health services for children and adolescents are hard to find, Herbert A. Schreier's department serves a large number of inner-city youth, accomplishing impressive results. In Chapter Eight, he discusses ways to make therapy work with this difficult population, including reliance on more than one therapeutic modality and creative utilization of the services of trainees.

Carl I. Cohen, in Chapter Nine, disagrees with the notion that the elderly are not accessible to psychotherapy. He presents a social analysis of the plight of the elderly and then, like most of the contributors to this sourcebook, suggests that the way to adapt psychotherapy to the needs of this population is to bring that social analysis into the therapeutic encounter. Greater insight is attained, and it becomes possible to plan for both psychological and social interventions.

Similarly, Lee Schore points out, in Chapter Ten, that the underutilization of mental health services by blue-collar workers has something to do with providers' failure to understand fully the plight of the workers and to provide relevant services. Drawing on her vast experience in providing mental health services to working-class communities, she suggests ways to adapt psychodynamic principles in working with this population.

Cutbacks in resources have prompted the establishment of time limits. Meanwhile, with deinstitutionalization and the arrival of severely disturbed and dually diagnosed clients in the community mental health system, clinicians are required to treat more difficult cases within these briefer and stricter time limits. In the final chapter, I discuss this trend, suggest a clinical strategy that is sometimes useful, and comment on the need for clinicians to speak out if we are to avert some of the trend's potentially detrimental consequences.

Terry A. Kupers
Editor

References

Anthony, W. A., and Liberman, R. P. "The Practice of Psychiatric Rehabilitation: Historical, Conceptual, and Research Base." *Schizophrenia Bulletin*, 1986, *12*(4), 542–559.

Bachrach, L. L., and Lamb, H. R. "What Have We Learned from Deinstitutionalization?" *Psychiatric Annals*, 1989, *19* (1), 12–21.

Brown, V. B., Ridgeley, M., Pepper, B., Levine, I. S., and Ryglewicz, H. "The Dual Crisis: Mental Illness and Substance Abuse." *American Psychologist*, 1989, *44* (3), 565–569.

Cutler, D., and Lefley, H. (eds.) "Training Professionals to Work with the Chronically Mentally Ill." *Community Mental Health Journal*, 1988, *11* (1), entire issue.

Danley, K. S., and Anthony, W. A. "The Choose-Get-Keep Model: Serving Severely Psychiatrically Disabled People." *American Rehabilitation*, October–December, 1987, pp. 6–11.

Glass, L. L., Katz, H. M., Schnitzer, R. D., Knapp, P. H., Frank, A. F., and Gunderson, J. G. "Psychotherapy of Schizophrenia: An Empirical Investigation of the Relationship of Process to Outcome." *American Journal of Psychiatry*, 1989, *146* (5), 603–608.

Harris, M., and Bachrach, L. L. (eds.). *Clinical Case Management.* New Directions for Mental Health Services, no. 40. San Francisco: Jossey-Bass, 1988.

Karon, B. P., and Vandenbos, G. R. *Psychotherapy of Schizophrenia: The Treatment of Choice.* New York: Aronson, 1981.

Kupers, T. A. *Public Therapy: The Practice of Psychotherapy in the Public Mental Health Clinic.* New York: Free Press, 1981.

Lamb, H. R. *Treating the Long-Term Mentally Ill.* San Francisco: Jossey-Bass, 1982.

Lamb, H. R. "One-to-One Relationships with the Long-Term Mentally Ill: Issues in Training Professionals." *Community Mental Health Journal,* 1988, *24* (4), 328–337.

Pepper, B., Kirshner, M., and Ryglewicz, H. "The Young Adult Chronic Patient: Overview of a Population." *Hospital and Community Psychiatry,* 1981, *32,* 463–469.

Solomon, P., Davis, J., and Gordon, B. "Discharged State Hospital Patients' Characteristics and Use of Aftercare: Effect on Community Tenure." *American Journal of Psychiatry,* 1984, *141* (12), 1566–1570.

Solomon, P., and Doll, W. "The Varieties of Readmission: The Case Against the Use of Recidivism Rates as a Measure of Program Effectiveness." *American Journal of Orthopsychiatry,* 1979, *4,* 230–239.

Stein, L. I., and Test, M. A. (eds.). *The Training in Community Living Model: A Decade of Experience.* New Directions for Mental Health Services, no. 26. San Francisco: Jossey-Bass, 1985.

Test, M. A., and Stein, L. I. "Community Treatment of the Chronic Patient: Research Overview." *Schizophrenia Bulletin,* 1978, *4,* 350–364.

Torrey, E. F. "Continuous-Treatment Teams in the Care of the Chronic Mentally Ill." *Hospital and Community Psychiatry,* 1986, *37,* 1243–1247.

Terry A. Kupers practices psychiatry in Oakland, California, is on the faculty of The Wright Institute in Berkeley, and is a consultant to several community mental health agencies.

The practice of psychotherapy must change in order to remain relevant to public mental health systems of the 1990s.

Psychotherapy and Community Support: Community Mental Health Systems in Transition

Gale G. Bataille

Psychotherapy, including long-term, insight-oriented therapy, can make a difference in the lives of poor and working-class adults, children, and families. But in this era of underfunded public mental health services, many are questioning the advisability of providing insight-oriented psychotherapy in the public sector. Mental health system administrators are telling clinicians to terminate long-term cases and to make room in their schedules to see more new patients. Clinicians are told to concentrate their practice on assessment, crisis intervention, brief therapy, and group psychotherapy. Therapy services are increasingly targeted to the seriously mentally ill population to the exclusion of others in need. In some cases, clinicians fight the implementation of the new priorities with the appeal: "Save psychotherapy for poor people." Meanwhile, in systems across the country, planners, administrators, and ultimately, elected officials are confronted with hard choices. It is estimated that funding nationally is less than 50 percent of what is necessary to care for the seriously mentally disabled in the community (Parrish, 1989; Stroul, 1989). Long-term individual psychotherapy requires a large staff and great expense. When budgets shrink, it is viewed as the item to cut. When clinicians protest, administrators may dismiss their concerns, believing that the clinicians are merely clinging to old and familiar work assignments and are resistant to learning new skills, such as brief therapy, group therapy, or case management.

When the dialogue between administrators and clinicians becomes polarized, the question is reduced to a choice between psychodynamic therapy for all people and a paraprofessional psychosocial model for management of the most dysfunctional patients. Clinicians who wish to continue what is essentially a private-practice model of psychotherapy in the public clinic argue that psychotherapy is practiced by professionals who support real change and growth for clients, including those who are the most disturbed. The alternative, case management and community support programs that emphasize psychosocial rehabilitation, merely represent the mechanistic management of patients' lives by paraprofessionals. The improvement in daily living skills brought about through psychosocial rehabilitation is valued by these clinicians, but is seen as less important than the intrapsychic change that only insight-oriented psychotherapy can bring about.

Of course, I have vastly simplified the argument. But in my encounters with outpatient clinicians who oppose many of the changes that are occurring in public mental health systems, I have found there to be a lack of recognition of the complex psychodynamic intervention skills required for the effective practice of clinical case management and psychosocial rehabilitation. I believe the controversy about the shift from long-term psychotherapy in the public clinic to a community support model is fueled by misconceptions and an incomplete analysis of the complex forces driving changes in federal, state, and local systems. And I believe that there is a key role for well-trained psychotherapists in the mental health system of the future—assuming that therapists can adapt their therapeutic approaches to new systems of care.

In this chapter, I will identify several of the trends that will shape public mental health care in the 1990s. I will comment on how and why the practice of psychotherapy must evolve in order to remain relevant, and finally, I will describe the kind of training that is needed in order to staff mental health systems in transition and the place that psychodynamic principles should have in the curriculum.

Four Trends in Public Mental Health Services for the 1990s

Rationed Care: Services to the Most Disabled. Public-sector mental health services are undergoing a profound transformation. Consider the recent (1986) federal legislation, Public Law 99-660, which mandates that states submit plans for identifying and serving specified priority populations—seriously and persistently mentally ill adults, homeless, dually diagnosed substance-abusing mentally disabled persons, and seriously emotionally disordered children. Federal Medicaid funding is tied to compliance with this law's requirements. This legislation offers a progressive vision of a mental health system that promotes the rights of seriously mentally disabled individuals to "live, learn, and work in environments of their choice" (Anthony and Liberman, 1986, p. 542). It begins to redress the twenty years of neglect that occurred in the name of deinstitutionalization and community mental health. Unfortunately, Public Law 99-660 also represents a federal retrenchment from the 1960s vision of comprehensive mental health care for all citizens. It is an acknowledgment and rationalization of an inadequate, two-class health care system in a nation where human services continue to be eroded in the name of deficit reduction. Thus, the shift away from long-term psychotherapy in public clinics reflects this acknowledgment of the erosion of care, while the argument that less staff-intensive treatment modalities offer just as much benefit is part of the rationalization.

Public Law 99-660 and the initiatives passed by those states viewed as leaders in developing systems of care—Ohio, Rhode Island, Wisconsin, and Michigan among them—explicitly target services to the most acutely or seriously mentally disabled populations. The exclusion of other populations who were previously served by community mental health centers is a source of conflict for many providers. The newly defined priority populations include those mentally disabled persons whose problems are exacerbated by substance use and abuse. It is estimated that over 50 percent of the mentally disabled (ages eighteen to forty-five) are dually diagnosed (Ridgely, Osher, and Talbott, 1987). All too often these patients fail to respond to treatment, or they resist it and are abandoned by the public sector as unmotivated and untreatable. Increasingly, these individuals populate state and county jails (Jemelka, Trupin, and Chiles, 1989).

There are also new populations to serve. As the baby-boom generation ages, there will be an increasingly large cohort of persons with mental problems linked to aging and to drug abuse. The number of seriously emotionally disturbed children, including those placed in foster care and out of home care, is rising dramatically. Some geographic areas are significantly impacted by migrant and immigrant populations suffering from posttraumatic stress syndrome and cultural dislocations. The victims of AIDS exhibit both psychological dysfunctions and organic dementias. These populations present both acute and chronic problems that require specialized intervention and language skills not readily available from professionals in most mental health systems.

There are ways to adapt the practice of psychotherapy to these new exigencies. There are psychotherapists who are committed to working with the seriously mentally ill, and their skills are needed in community support and in in-home intervention programs. It is only relatively recently that therapists have specialized in assessing and treating elders,and only now are strategies appearing for psychotherapy with AIDS sufferers.

There is a pressing need for practitioners who can provide culturally relevant and sensitive services to ethnic minorities. With each new population to serve, therapists have a contribution to make.

The Growth of Consumer Advocacy. The National Alliance for the Mentally Ill (NAMI) is one of the fastest-growing consumer advocacy groups in the country with a current membership of over 80,000. Congressional testimony during hearings on Public Law 99-660 underscores the political strength of this organization. This self-help movement was energized by the anger of families who felt blamed by mental health professionals for the psychopathology of their mentally ill relatives. They felt that community mental health centers neglected the needsof the most disabled patients who were shunted from the back wardto the back alley. While the priority of NAMI remains biomedical research, the organization has become increasingly supportive of the development of a range of community support services that are psychosocial in emphasis.

Similar to NAMI in the way they evolved, though less politically powerful, are the national and state networks of direct mental health consumers. Organizations such as the National Alliance of Mental Patients and the National Mental Health Consumers' Association emphasize rights advocacy, the provision of client-oriented and client-operated voluntary services, self-help, and peer support as well as political action.

Organizations of families of the mentally ill and direct-consumer groups have significant ideological differences. However, they have allied to advocate for common concerns, such as greater availability of community support services and an end to discrimination against the mentally ill in housing, jobs, and education. Both the family and the direct-consumer movements question the effectiveness of psychotherapy for psychiatrically disabled populations and tend to support alternative models of care. The therapist's skills must be expanded to encompass and support the positive contributions of these rapidly organizing constituencies. Sometimes, it is the therapeutic sensibility that permits one to work through tensions between mental health providers and consumers. And perhaps, if therapists begin to listen to and value the expressed interests and needs of consumers and families of the mentally ill, the consumers and families will not be so hostile to the inclusion of therapy in the range of services offered by mental health systems.

New Forms of Involuntary Treatment. The criminal justice system has become a parallel system of psychiatric care. It is estimated that between 8 and 20 percent of incarcerated adults suffer from a major mental disorder (Jemelka, Trupin, and Chiles, 1989). In California, during the 1988–89 fiscal year, the only new mental health funding was for a psychiatric unit in the prison system. Meanwhile, programs of community-based involuntary care are developing for pretrial diversion, as well as for probationers, parolees, and mentally disordered offenders.

A number of states (including Washington, North Carolina, and Massachusetts) have instituted involuntary outpatient care for patients who suffer from a serious mental disorder, require multiple hospitalizations, and are noncompliant. The homeless mentally disabled and substance-abusing mentally disabled populations are disturbingly visible to the public. This visibility creates pressure for mandatory treatment and an abandonment of some of the civil rights protections gained in the past twenty years. At the same time, the public seems unwilling to pay the costs of mandatory treatment. The number of public-sector psychiatric beds and the funding for community treatment continue to decrease.

Public-sector mental health workers are required to move between the roles of supportive therapist and agent of the state with the power to confine a mentally ill person involuntarily in a jail or psychiatric hospital. These contradictory roles, the helper and the jailer, have always been present in psychiatry and in community mental health programs, but the contradictions are intensified when more uncooperative clients are served by the mental health system. And this trend wil become still more troubling if additional resources are not provided for the psychiatrically disabled in the 1990s. Psychotherapists have an important contribution to make here, but they face a real challenge: They must adapt the practice of therapy to the less voluntary setting while preserving the therapist's role as helper.

A Shift in Emphasis from Outpatient Clinics to Community Support Programs. A detailed discussion of this shift is beyond the scope of this chapter; however, I will mention several principles that are critically important to the changing practice of psychotherapy. These principles, discussed extensively in *Toward a Model Plan* (Parrish and Lieberman, 1987) and in the work of William Anthony and others (Anthony and Blanch, 1989) at the Center for Psychiatric Rehabilitation at Boston University, include the following:

- A consumer-centered approach emphasizing the rights of the psychiatrically disabled to "live, learn, and work" in environments of their choosing
- A focus on providing services in the client's natural environment with the type and intensity of support varying according to the client's level of need
- An emphasis on client goals and capacity rather than on psychopathology
- A commitment to a skills-based approach to services with the recognition that for some psychiatrically disabled persons, skills learned in one environment may not be easily transferable to another
- A recognition that services must be integrated and centered on the patient rather than on the program.

In some mental health systems, community support and social rehabilitation programs function largely in isolation from outpatient therapy services. This lack of integration among practices is dysfunctional for both the clients and the system. An understanding of psychodynamics and interpersonal change processes can enhance the rehabilitation approach. In well-functioning systems, these practices are not compartmentalized but rather are applied flexibly, depending on the particular needs and circumstances of each client.

Needed: A Multifaceted and Adaptable Psychotherapy

The art of psychotherapy, including the use of a relationship to support intrapsychic and interpersonal growth, can and should remain relevant to public mental health practice. Psychoanalysts had to adapt their methods to the exigencies of war during World War II and had to adapt to the advent of psychotropic medications in the 1950s. Today's public therapist is again at a critical juncture, facing a need for innovations in technique. Kupers (1981), for example, claims that the therapist must be willing to leave the clinic and visit the patient at home, in the hospital, or in prison and that it is sometimes therapeutic for him or her to act as the client's advocate during a disability hearing or court date.

Therapy, once practiced exclusively in an office or hospital setting, must now expand to become environmental. Therapeutic interventions must be woven into the tapestry of clients' lives. The therapist must know how the client lives; this often requires visits to the home or sessions conducted there. The therapist must address the client's problems at work or at school; this may require advocacy or collaboration with other service providers, such as the union steward or school officials. And the treatment must include help in relating to others, which might mean bringing some of those others into the treatment. The therapist must be able to move and adapt flexibly within a range of roles and practice methods, as advocate, teacher, group facilitator, family educator, resource developer, family therapist, and so on. The intervention might occur at the work site, in a community residential care facility, in the client's apartment, at school, or in a restaurant, as well as in the clinic. The type of therapeutic intervention might be individual, group, or family. It might be supportive, deeply probing, highly directive, educational, or consultative. And therapy might take the form of crisis intervention, brief therapy, or longer-term psychotherapy. The psychotherapist must be able and willing to do a little of each, as indicated in any particular instance.

How are psychotherapeutic principles useful in work with families and consumer groups? Without blaming and labeling family members, therapists can act as consultants and educators, essentially collaborating with families to develop coping strategies for living with and caring for a seriously disabled relative. The therapist, drawing on a clinical background, can explain the extent of a family member's disability as well as his or her capabilities and potentialities. The role of educator and family consultant is not an alternative to that of therapist; rather, it demands a high degree of therapeutic experience and skill. And these consultative approaches with families have proved effective (Kanter, 1985; Hatfield, 1984).

An understanding of interpersonal dynamics and group process can also be used to support the self-help and peer-support activities of direct mental health consumers. A growing number of services are staffed and operated by consumers. These include housing programs, drop-in centers, rights protection programs, and small businesses. Providers must support and learn from the program models and accomplishments of direct consumers. As in the case of families, therapists can act as teachers and consultants, sharing their clinical knowledge and their therapeutic skills. Here it is important for therapists to stay in the consultant role and not act as group leaders, as the leadership must come from the consumers themselves. An understanding of the healing power of self-help groups may be a prerequisite for the therapist to be effective in this kind of supportive role.

Finally, it is critical that mental health systems develop effective treatment interventions with substance-abusing psychiatrically disabled individuals, given their high prevalence rates and high cost to society (Ridgely, Osher, and Talbott, 1987; Brown and others, 1989). Clinicians, administrators, and policy makers must join together in order to have real impact (Bataille, 1989). Treatment approaches and programs must draw on and integrate the knowledge and skills of psychotherapy, chemical dependency treatment, self-help groups (such as Alcoholics Anonymous), and the mental health consumer movement. The dually diagnosed are a challenge to the mental health system. Compartmentalization in programs and methods of practice, rigid definitions of target populations, and some regulatory restrictions must be dropped if there is to be an effective response. Again, therapists working with the dually diagnosed need to become flexible and to develop new intervention repertories. For instance, it is no longer acceptable to refuse therapy to a client solely because that client abuses alcohol or drugs. At the same time, insight-oriented psychotherapy with an intoxicated client is a waste of time.

I have mentioned only a few examples of how psychotherapy will need to change in order to be relevant to mental health services in the nineties. If clinical staff are to function effectively in their new and evolving roles, a dramatically expanded commitment must be made to training and staff development.

Training and Staff Development

Public therapists must increase the range of their intervention capabilities. When they resist innovations in the provision of mental health services, it is due in large part to insufficient attention to their training for new roles. In spite of federal legislation targeting specific populations and advances in techniques for the provision of community support services, clinical work with the seriously mentally ill is still a low priority in most graduate programs for mental health professionals (Hargrove and Spaulding, 1988). A hopeful sign is that some programs are currently developing specialized tracks that focus on public-sector needs.

The private practice of psychotherapy, with an emphasis on psychodynamic individual and family therapy, continues to be viewed as the highest career goal by many practitioners. I have had numerous conversations with therapists in the system where I work who state that they are not trained or interested in working as clinical case managers in a community support model and that they will resist doing so because they believe that their current practice is making a difference in people's lives. Other clinicians publicly acknowledge their lack of training and experience in crisis intervention, brief therapy, or group therapy with seriously mentally disabled clients. Thus, they are ill equipped to provide the types of therapeutic interventions that are likely to be offered in the public sector in the next decade.

A 1987 survey (Daniels and Goodrick, 1987) of state mental health training and resource development needs identified staff investment in current programs and methods as a major barrier to systems change. A recent national forum to promote training of professionals for more effective work with the seriously mentally disabled identified the following training and staff development needs: motivating graduate program faculty and administrators to focus on this population, developing curricula that reflect current research and practice, and developing continuing education for working professionals (Lefley, Bernheim, and Goldman, 1989). Any graduate program in mental health that aims to teach the skills and methods that will serve their graduates well in public-sector practice must include in the curriculum the principles of psychotherapy, as well as methods for adapting psychodynamic principles to the tasks of the new public therapist. The same principles and methods can be taught, in the form of staff training or continuing professional education, to practitioners in the field.

Meanwhile, therapists who cling to traditional individual-oriented and office-based practice will be displaced from the public sector. Mental health program administrators and staff must become change experts in the next decade. This transformation in the public sector will be limited by a continuing poverty of resources, but there is also real potential for the development of services that meet the needs of consumers. One can hope that psychotherapists will make important contributions to the process of change and in that process will learn or invent new ways to adapt psychotherapy to contemporary problems. Our ability to create a responsive public mental health system is linked to our ability as administrators and direct service providers to plan together for change and to hear and respect the perspectives and goals of our clients and their families.

References

Anthony, W. A., and Blanch, A. "Research on Community Support Services: What Have We Learned?" *Psychosocial Rehabilitation Journal,* 1989, *12* (3), 55–82.

Anthony, W. A., and Liberman, R. P. "The Practice of Psychiatric Rehabilitation: Historical, Conceptual, and Research Base." *Schizophrenia Bulletin,* 1986, *12* (4), 542–559.

Bataille, G. G. "The Multiply Diagnosed: A Challenge to the System—Recommendations for Improving Services to Substance-Abusing Mentally Disabled Persons." Paper presented at the California Conference of Local Mental Health Directors, Burlingame, California, February 9, 1989.

Brown, V. B., Ridgely, M. S., Pepper, B., Levine, I. S., and Ryglewicz, H. "The Dual Crisis: Mental Illness and Substance Abuse." *American Psychologist,* 1989, *44* (3), 565–569.

Daniels, L., and Goodrick, D. "Survey of Training Needs: State Mental Health Agency Mental Health System Strategic Planning." Washington, D.C.: Mental Health Strategic Planning Project, Alpha Center for Health Planning, 1987.

Hatfield, A. *Coping with Mental Illness in the Family: A Family Guide.* Washington, D.C.: National Alliance for the Mentally Ill, 1984.

Jemelka, R., Trupin, E., and Chiles, J. "The Mentally Ill in Prisons: A Review." *Hospital and Community Psychiatry,* 1989, *40,* 486–489.

Kanter, J. "Case Management of the Young Adult Chronic Patient: A Clinical Perspective." In J. Kanter (ed.), *Clinical Issues in Treating the Chronically Mentally Ill.* New Directions for Mental Health Services, no. 27. San Francisco: Jossey-Bass, 1985.

Kupers, T. A. *Public Therapy: The Practice of Psychotherapy in the Public Mental Health Clinic.* New York: Free Press, 1981.

Lefley, H. P., Bernheim, K. F., and Goldman, C. R. "Conference Report: National Forum for Educating Mental Health Professionals to Work with the Seriously Mentally Ill and Their Families." *Hospital and Community Psychiatry,* 1989, *40,* 460–470.

Parrish, J. "The Long Journey Home: Accomplishing the Mission of the Community Support Movement." *Psychosocial Rehabilitation Journal,* 1989, *12* (3), 107–124.

Parrish, J., and Lieberman, M. *Toward a Model Plan for a Comprehensive, Community-Based Mental Health System.* Rockville, Md.: National Institute of Mental Health, 1987.

Ridgely, M. S., Osher, S. C., and Talbott, J. A. *Chronically Mentally Ill Young Adults with Substance Abuse Problems: Treatment and Training Issues.* Baltimore: University of Maryland Mental Health Policy Studies, University of Maryland, 1987.

Stroul, B. "Community Support Systems for Persons with Long-Term Mental Illness: A Conceptual Framework." *Psychosocial Rehabilitation Journal,* 1989, *12* (3), 9–26.

Gale G. Bataille is deputy director of the Alcohol/Drug Abuse/ Mental Abuse Division of the Health Services Department in Contra Costa County, California. She has worked as a therapist, planner, program developer, and manager in public mental health programs for the past twenty years, both in a state hospital and in community programs.

Clinical case management can facilitate the chronically mentally ill patient's ability to function effectively in the community. Case examples demonstrate the use of psychodynamic principles in the delivery of community mental health services.

The Uses of Therapy in Case Management

Cheryl M. Bryan

Case management initially evolved out of a need to coordinate community aftercare services for the chronically mentally ill. Since that time, many attempts have been made to conceptualize the role of the case manager and the function of case management services in a way that would transcend the mere coordination of systems (Lamb, 1980; Kanter, 1989). While the actual practice of case management varies from agency to agency, the functions of the case manager are generally thought to include assessment, planning, linking, monitoring, and advocacy. With this in mind, many mental health workers think of case management as merely providing managerial services. Too little thought is given to the clinical and therapeutic aspects of this particular type of intervention.

Lamb (1980) suggests that the case manager should be more than just a "broker of services" and should be the patient's primary therapist. Harris and Bergman (1987) state that case management is not only a means for coordinating systems and services but should also be viewed as a distinct mode of therapy in itself. They base this idea on the fact that it is generally the case manager who collects data from a wide variety of sources and can develop the most in-depth and comprehensive knowledge and understanding of a patient. The other individual components of the system each have a very limited view of the patient, often defined by a specific form of treatment. For example, the vocational rehabilitation counselor knows the patient's vocational strengths and weaknesses, while the psychiatrist focuses specifically on the patient's response to medication and side effects. The case manager is in the best position to assess the patient's overall strengths, weaknesses, and capabilities.

Although many writers have attempted to define the role of the case manager and the functions of case management services, little attention has been paid to the principles of case management as a therapeutic intervention. While the case manager does not have to be a therapist in order to provide case management services, I would like to illustrate how my training in psychodynamic theory has been incorporated in my work as a case manager. In this chapter, I will first discuss case management as a particular type of therapeutic intervention, focusing primarily on the application of psychodynamic principles in working with the chronically mentally ill, and then I will suggest how psychodynamic principles can be used in restructuring the delivery of services in the community mental health system.

Psychotherapy and the Chronically Mentally Ill

Chronically mentally ill patients suffer from many emotional deficits. They are highly vulnerable to stress and anxiety. They have difficulty coping with the daily demands of life. They often lack a stable identity and secure sense of self. They have a difficult time establishing and maintaining meaningful interpersonal relationships. It is no surprise that these patients experience a great deal of difficulty adjusting to life in the community after their release from a mental health institution.

Individuals who have been identified as needing case management services generally meet the following criteria: They have had at least two psychiatric hospitalizations in the last six months (or three psychiatric hospitalizations in the last twelve months), or they may be high users of psychiatric emergency services (showing up in crisis a few times a month); they suffer from a severe and chronic mental disorder; and they have failed to link with community outpatient services or are unable to follow through with outpatient services (by keeping scheduled appointments or taking medications, for example).

Psychotherapy is believed to bring about internal growth and change with a resultant increase in the capacity to cope with the daily stresses of life. Often clinicians trained to do psychodynamic psychotherapy are discouraged when their efforts to use psychodynamic principles with the chronic patient seem unsuccessful. Many clinicians then feel that the chronically mentally ill patient cannot benefit from psychotherapy and can only benefit from supportive therapy and/or psychopharmacological interventions (Minkoff, 1987). Case management services are thought to affect only the patient's external world without facilitating any internal growth or change, and many clinicians are reluctant to engage in the practice of case management. Effective clinical case management, however, can facilitate the patient's capacity to cope and function more effectively in his or her day-to-day life. In psychodynamic terms, this occurs when the patient is able to internalize the role of the case manager and the functions of case management.

While it is true that the practice of "traditional" (insight-oriented) psychodynamic psychotherapy is not particularly effective with the severely mentally ill, an understanding of psychopathology, psychodynamic principles, and the stages of human development is essential for making appropriate therapeutic interventions. Chronic mental illness does not preclude the presence of underlying conflicts accompanied by defenses aimed at helping the individual cope more effectively with these conflicts. The defenses utilized by the chronic patient are quite primitive. These generally consist of denial, projection, projective identification, and splitting. One must pay particular attention to the transference and countertransference issues that will emerge during the course of treatment.

The Role of Case Manager. The initial role played by the case manager is, out of necessity, a managerial one. It involves providing the patient with concrete assistance, which may include finding a place for the patient to live once he or she leaves the hospital, helping him or her obtain financial entitlements to provide a means of support, helping him or her find structured daily activities to minimize social isolation, arranging for follow-up medication appointments, and so on. The patient's current response to the case manager will be based on distorted images of past relationships. No matter how hard case managers attempt to be sensitive and empathic to the needs of the individual patient, they become receptacles for the distorted projections elicited by the implicitly parental functions of their managerial role (Searles, 1982). The case manager may be idealized as omnipotent and all-loving or devalued as stupid, unfeeling, and ineffectual (Kanter, 1985). In order to make an appropriate therapeutic intervention, the case manager must understand the conflicting conscious and unconscious motives of the severely mentally ill patient. There is often a conflict between the patient's yearnings for both independence and dependence and a fear of having a separate identity or of losing one's boundaries and merging with the case manager.

The Reenactment of Emotional Conflicts. Both the severely mentally ill and higher-functioning neurotic patients become involved in the reenactment of distressing emotional conflicts (repetition compulsion). It is often easier for the clinician to understand and interpret behavior that seems well within the "normal" range of experiences. Behaviors that seem more bizarre or inappropriate can elicit uncomfortable, negative countertransference responses on the part of the clinician. Clinicians may have a harder time relating to the patient and knowing how and when to intervene. Knowledge of the individual patient's early family history, of traumatic events that may have interfered with the developmental growth process, of events that precipitated psychotic episodes, of current life circumstances, of how the individual handles losses, and so on becomes extremely helpful in beginning to understand what is being reenacted in the treatment, and this knowledge can help the clinician recognize possible transference issues. Clinicians must also be aware of the impact that their behaviors and actions can have on the patient, even when the patient is not always able to verbalize his or her feelings.

In addition, clinicians need to recognize that the mental health system may, by the very nature of its structure, be countertherapeutic. For example, the length of stay in a residential treatment facility is limited to a few months. Many severely emotionally disturbed patients have just begun to develop a trusting relationship with their counselor or therapist at the end of their stay. Terminating this important relationship often triggers a regressive or psychotic episode. An understanding of psychodynamic principles can help the case manager establish an important connection with the patient. This may be the one enduring relationship, which helps the patient cope with issues of separation and loss.

Since case management involves the development of a close working relationship between the case manager and the patient, there is always an opportunity for identification and imitation of the behaviors of the case manager, and this can mark the beginning of therapeutic growth (Harris and Bergman, 1987).

The following case examples from my own experience illustrate these points.

The Case of Ms. M. Ms. M., a young adult, was diagnosed as a paranoid schizophrenic. When she first began coming to the clinic, she was unable to stay for longer than ten minutes and would sit as far away from me (the case manager) as possible. She would leave the room for short periods and then return. She carried a day pack that contained some changes of clothing and also a can of Lysol spray. She would ritualistically spray everything she touched and would spray the room when she left. She was experiencing auditory hallucinations. She indicated that the voices said bad things about her and would comment specifically about her body odor. She frequently moved from one hotel to the next because of "people standing outside my door talking about the way I smell." (It should be noted that no body odor was evident.) She refused to take medication and did not want to believe that she had any kind of mental illness.

Our initial sessions felt frustrating to me. Ms. M. talked little. When she did, it was simply to report another incident at her hotel and her plans to move. My comments or questions led to Ms. M.'s stating that she had to leave the room and would be right back. I felt that my most useful interventions were in arranging for Ms. M. to participate in a vocational rehabilitation program or day treatment. She would begin these classes but would inevitably drop out because she again thought people were talking about her offensive body odor. Ms. M. indicated that she felt she had no other option but to leave when people said bad things about her. During one of our sessions, Ms. M. stated, "You know, sometimes you smell bad." And she wanted to know if she had hurt my feelings by telling me this. We then had a brief discussion about body odors and noted that people's feelings can be hurt if someone tells them they smell bad. Following this session, Ms. M. came in to report proudly that she had again heard someone in her class saying something bad about how she smelled, but she was not going to leave the class. This time she felt she had a right to be there just like everybody else. Our sessions began to last longer, Ms. M. began staying in her classes longer, she moved less frequently, and she stopped spraying the office.

My vacations were soon noted, however, to trigger regressive episodes on the part of the patient. Whenever I was on vacation, the auditory hallucinations increased, and Ms. M.'s behavior became more influenced by paranoid delusions. To help Ms. M. gain some insight into this phenomenon, I commented about how unsafe the world seemed to her whenever I was going to be away, linking this with the way her "voices" would get louder and her fear greater. We began to talk about some concrete ways she could take care of herself while I was away. One of the most effective methods the patient found for coping with my absence was to have some "transitional object" such as my business card or something from my desk that she could hold until I returned. This helped her hold on to me and keep me with her even though I was absent. This suggests that developmentally the patient was unable to maintain object constancy and needed help believing that the case manager continued to exist in the case manager's absence. Ms. M. was soon willing to recognize that the 'voices" might not be real and was willing to try taking medication to see if they would go away.

Family History. A brief review of the patient's early family history provides some insight into the dynamics being reenacted in our sessions. The patient had been given up for adoption when she was an infant. Her adoptive mother was killed in a car accident, and the patient was then raised by her grandmother (the adoptive mother's mother). When the patient was in her midteens, her grandmother died of what may have been the complications of Alzheimer's disease, and the patient blamed herself for not taking better care of her grandmother. The patient began having psychotic symptoms soon after the death of her grandmother.

Discussion. This patient suffered many serious losses and unconsciously believed that somehow there was something so offensive about her that it could destroy or kill anyone or anything she cared about. She deeply wanted to be dependent on someone but was fearful of becoming too attached to anyone. To protect herself and others, she would remove herself from the situation, which left her feeling isolated and lonely. What became therapeutic for this patient was the case manager's ability not only to recognize the unconscious conflicts but also to make sure the patient learned that the case manager would not be destroyed by the offensive odors or "insults" from the patient. The patient could leave the room, come back, and see that the case manager was still there. When the patient, via projective identification, stated that it was the case manager that had a bad odor, the case manager did not leave or ask the patient to leave, but stayed to discuss the issue and the associated feelings. The patient, in identifying with the case manager, was then able to emulate the case manager's reaction, thus enabling her to begin introjecting a less destructive image of herself. This allowed her to become more involved in relationships with other people and to follow through on participation in her day-treatment program.

The Case of Mr. C. Mr. C., a borderline patient, had a number of short-term psychiatric hospitalizations for suicidal threats and ideation. Socially isolated and fearful of living alone, he was discharged to a psychiatric halfway house. Here he could stay for a maximum of three months. Soon after arriving at the halfway house, Mr. C. began exhibiting typical "borderline traits." He was demanding, stubborn, hostile, sarcastic, and devaluing of the staff and the treatment program. When the staff attempted to set limits with him, he accused them of abusing him and trying to force him to leave the program. The staff quickly became divided on whether or not Mr. C. could benefit from being in a halfway house and considered terminating him from the program. After pushing most of the house rules and staff to the limit, Mr. C. settled into the routine of the program. As he approached the termination phase and began to prepare for transition into a cooperative, independent-living household, his borderline characteristics began to escalate. He had a hard time adjusting to his new household. He was again exhibiting anger, hostility, and impulsivity; he devalued the staff, threatened suicide, and was eventually rehospitalized. On discharge from the hospital, Mr. C. was ambivalent about returning to his current household. He blamed the staff for hospitalizing him and trying to get rid of him, and he then decided to leave the program.

As his case manager, I met with Mr. C. weekly throughout these transitions. Initially, he seemed to establish a positive, idealized transference toward me. He saw me as the person who would take care of him and protect him. When I could not "fix" things for him with the staff of his current household, I too became the recipient of his rageful devaluation. One day, before he stormed out of my office, I attempted to validate the fact that his feelings had been hurt by the way he felt he had been treated by everyone, and I indicated that I knew he was angry with me for not taking better care of him. I also indicated that I was still interested in working with him. I pointed out some of the successful work we had done together and expressed my hope that he would still want to work with me at some point. He left the office in a huff, slamming the door. Two weeks later, he called, very apologetic, and asked me if I would still be willing to work with him.

Family History. Mr. C. was the youngest of three siblings. His parents did not get along well and often engaged in verbal and physical fighting. The patient indicated that he was also beaten by his parents. Mr. C. indicated that the teachers at school knew what was going on, because he often showed up at school with bruises, but nobody intervened. His father left home when Mr. C. was thirteen years old. His mother died when the patient was sixteen. Mr. C.'s older sister then took care of him, but he left home one year later. He indicated that he had always felt unwanted and tended to live a solitary and isolated existence.

Discussion. Mr. C.'s adult behavior demonstrates a number of ways in which he is reenacting earlier interpersonal family dynamics. Transference issues emerged early in the treatment with Mr. C. experiencing the case manager as the omnipotent, nurturing, and all-loving good parent. But as his conflicts with dependency and his fears of being abused and abandoned emerged, the good parent was soon replaced by the bad parent. Mr. C.'s attempts to defend against his fears of dependency and abandonment (via projection, devaluation, and so on) produced strong negative countertransference feelings on the part of the case manager and other mental health workers involved in his treatment. It was important for the case manager to be able to recognize and understand the patient's conflictual dilemma and not act punitively on the negative countertransference feelings that the patient clearly evoked. The case manager needed to remain consistently empathic and interested in the patient, while at the same time setting firm limits. This allowed the patient to see that his behavior would not result in abandonment. Conversely, this patient needed to learn that "getting better" did not have to result in abandonment.

The mental health system, as it is currently established, was not particularly responsive to Mr. C.'s needs. The fact that all patients must keep transferring to new settings and readjusting to new staff and new programs is extremely stressful. The most well-adjusted individual would probably experience some anxiety at having to face new people, new settings, and new challenges again and again.

The Structure of the Community Mental Health System

In an attempt to respond to the needs of the chronically mentally ill patient, the community mental health system is composed of many different segments. Each segment focuses on a particular aspect of treatment. The length of stay in each program or facility varies and is subject to change each year based on funding. Inpatient hospitalizations at the local hospital may range from a seventy-two-hour evaluation to a two-week hospital stay. The patient may then be transferred to an acute diversion unit where he or she may stay for an average length of two weeks. Some patients may be placed in a halfway house where they may stay for up to three months. During this time, patients are expected to be involved in a number of groups and other forms of day treatment. Each program has its own rules and expectations, and patients who are considered problematic or noncompliant are terminated. This type of system overlooks the fact that the patients who are the most chronic users of community mental health programs are forced to undergo continual transitions that often trigger major regressive episodes.

It is unfortunate that the delivery of services in the community mental health system is so restricted by time limits. This structure creates difficulties for patients who have problems with separation and loss (which includes most of the chronically mentally ill). Psychodynamic principles and developmental theory point out that the process of growth and change occurs over a long period of time. For the severely mentally ill patient, this process will take even longer. In the future, programs should be designed to meet the psychological and developmental needs of the patient, rather than requiring patients to conform to a preestablished treatment format. Meanwhile, the case manager can provide continuity for the patient and can help minimize the patient's feelings of abandonment.

References

Harris, M., and Bergman, H. C. "Case Management with the Chronically Mentally Ill: A Clinical Perspective." *American Journal of Orthopsychiatry*, 1987, *57* (2), 296-302.

Kanter, J. "Case Management of the Young Adult Chronic Patient: A Clinical Perspective." In J. Kanter (ed.), *Clinical Issues in Treating the Chronically Mentally Ill*. New Directions for Mental Health Services, no. 27. San Francisco: Jossey-Bass, 1985.

Kanter, J. "Clinical Case Management: Definition, Principles, Components." *Hospital and Community Psychiatry*, 1989, *40* (4), 361-368.

Lamb, H. R. "Therapists—Case Managers: More Than Brokers of Service." *Hospital and Community Psychiatry*, 1980, *31*, 762-764.

Minkoff, K. "Resistance of Mental Health Professionals to Working with the Chronically Mentally Ill." In A. T. Meyerson (ed.), *Barriers to Treating the Chronic Mentally Ill*. New Directions for Mental Health Services, no. 33. San Francisco: Jossey-Bass, 1987.

Searles, H. "The Analyst as Manager of the Patient's Daily Life: Transference and Countertransference Dimensions of the Relationship." *International Journal of Psychoanalytic Psychotherapy*, 1982, *11*, 475-486.

Cheryl M. Bryan is staff psychologist and coordinator of clinical training for the Citywide Case Management Program in the Department of Psychiatry at the University of California, San Francisco. She is on the faculty of New College of California and maintains a private practice in San Francisco.

*In this age of deinstitutionalization and community-based
services for those suffering from chronic mental disorders,
mental health practitioners—both psychotherapists and
providers of other services—need to understand the
psychodynamics as well as the social realities of chronicity.*

Therapy and Chronicity

Richard Bloom

The need to apply a psychodynamic understanding of chronicity is
greater today than it has ever been. In the late 1970s and early 1980s,
clinicians in community mental health centers found themselves working
with large numbers of patients who had been recently deinstitutionalized.
The inpatient population in the United States went from 560,000 in 1955
to 116,000 last year (Bachrach and Lamb, 1989). The movement toward
community-based treatment was founded on the idea of preventing severe
mental disorders and chronicity (Lamb and Zusman, 1981). Programs
and treatment goals were explicitly directed toward dealing with the
dangers of institutionalized "patienthood." Social rehabilitation and reintegration into community life were goals that clinicians considered as
important as the treatment of the symptoms of psychopathological conditions (Zusman and Lamb, 1977). As time passed, the issue of preventing
or reversing chronicity was placed lower on the list of priorities. This
was partly due to the fact that outcome studies demonstrated that psychotherapy had limited lasting positive effect (Test and Stein, 1978), but
mainly the decreased interest in treating and preventing chronicity was a
direct effect of cutbacks in funding for clinical, social rehabilitative, and
other social services. Now, instead of spending sufficient time talking to
patients, understanding their problems and their psychodynamics, and
offering them enough psychotherapy and rehabilitation to help them
avoid the worst results of chronicity, overworked clinicians are more
likely to rely heavily on psychotropic medications. With less resources,
the outcomes for psychotherapy are, of course, worse. Even though we
are faced with an entire generation of patients who have deeply entrenched chronic conditions (Pepper, Kirshner, and Ryglewicz, 1981), the

New Directions for Mental Health Services, no. 46, Summer 1990 © Jossey-Bass Inc., Publishers prevention and reversal of chronicity is no longer an explicit priority for program planners, and it is fast disappearing from the dynamic formulation and treatment plans of clinicians in the public sector.

Of course, it is important to attend to the basic survival needs of our most disturbed patients and to their skills in daily living. But the prevention or reversal of chronicity—in however many cases this is still a realistic goal—cannot be accomplished without a deeper understanding of internal psychic processes and related issues of identity. Chronicity is a term that applies to the external circumstances of living as well as to the ways in which ego functions and a sense of self are structured and maintained (Zusman, 1966). According to the *Diagnostic and Statistical Manual of Mental Disorders* (DSM-III-R), a major mental illness is considered chronic in patients whose symptoms endure for a certain length of time. This is one use of the term. From a psychodynamic perspective, in particular from the perspective of an object-relations or ego psychology model, the symptoms of chronicity can be viewed as defensive maneuvers—that is, they represent the patient's regressed and desperate attempts to maintain a basic sense of existence and identity while coping with an external world that seems extremely threatening (Kupers, 1981). This psychodynamic perspective is not inconsistent with the interpretation offered by sociologists of deviance that chronicity is a reflection of socialization into the patient role in the institution (Goffman, 1961; Scheff, 1966). The psychodynamic perspective addresses the subjective experience while the sociological focuses on the objective or the external context. According to Lamb (1982), secondary symptoms of chronicity constitute a form of social disability in which the individual identifies with the sick role, characterized by social withdrawal, helplessness, and hopelessness. Treatment approaches that encourage passivity, helplessness, and dependency merely reinforce a seriously disturbed patient's perceptions of the external world as consisting of uncontrollable forces that act on the individual, who is merely an object with no power.

In spite of large mental health budget reductions, not all therapeutic, social rehabilitative, and support services have been eliminated. In the context of services that remain viable, providers often find it difficult to engage patients whose defenses have been hardened by years of chronicity. The lessons learned from psychotherapy with chronic patients can be applied in other settings. For instance, the ostensibly simple task of developing a therapeutic relationship—whether this be in therapy sessions or in the context of a day-treatment or halfway house program—becomes very arduous. Here is where it is crucial that the clinician understand the patient's psychodynamics, even if therapy is not the object. The clinician's understanding of the defensive uses of chronicity and the fragility of the chronic patient's identity helps in the process of "getting through" to the recipient of services, helps the provider transcend the client's negativism and "stuckness" at points along the way, and in many cases determines the success or failure of those services.

For instance, the clinician must understand why the patient experiences any mention of a change in life-style as incredibly threatening. The clinician's understanding of the patient's need to hold on to whatever meager sense of continuity there is in a very marginal life-style serves as an antidote to countertransference feelings of frustration, impatience, and hopelessness. One can hope that the clinician and the patient will spend enough time talking to develop some mutual understanding and to establish realistic treatment goals. Perhaps the clinician must be satisfied with some degree of loosening of chronic defenses so that the patient can avail himself or herself of some of the available resources; the clinician may need to let go of the expectation that there will be a dramatic shift in ego functioning and a radical change of life-style. Still, the clinician's understanding of the psychodynamics can help accomplish the more realistic goals.

I practice psychotherapy in a public mental health clinic and will present an example of my work with one patient. Others who work with similar patients, even though they do not practice what they would call psychotherapy, should be able to utilize the experience garnered from the conduct of therapy to understand the clients with whom they work and to devise effective strategies for helping their clients accomplish the program's goals.

The Case of Mr. D.

Mr. D., a fifty-two-year-old man, was brought into the community mental health clinic by his younger sister and his former wife. At first he was reluctant to come in, as if he had more to lose than to gain. He was quite withdrawn and somewhat disoriented and noncommunicative. He wore ragged, filthy clothing and appeared as "down and out" as could be. He was extremely depressed, and his thought processes were disordered, including poor reality testing. His hygiene was poor, and he exhibited some ritualistic behaviors. For instance, he would engage in a complicated process of positioning his knapsack carefully and then moving it and repositioning it three or four times before sitting down. However, he was capable of conducting a rational conversation, possessed a dry sense of humor, and showed signs of above-average intelligence.

Mr. D. was born and raised in a middle-class Caucasian family in the Bay Area. He suffered a first breakdown toward the end of his college days. He was able to work intermittently for the next ten years, but he has lived the life of a chronic unemployed patient since approximately 1975. At times he has been homeless, and there have been a number of hospitalizations and some sporadic outpatient therapy. He had refused to take medications for several years prior to arriving at the clinic. Both of his parents had died when they were in their mid sixties, and Mr. D. worried that he was becoming an old man.

After being evaluated, he was advised that he would be eligible for disability benefits from the Social Security Administration—Supplemental Security Income (SSI)—and he was invited to embark on a course of psychotherapy with me. With some coaxing from his relatives, he agreed to begin therapy. For months he let others bring him in for appointments, but he persistently rejected the idea of applying for Social Security (Disability) Insurance (SSI). He would say that he thought it would be better for him to "keep looking for a part-time job." It was this catchphrase that alerted me to the fact that he really did feel he was in danger of losing something about himself. Although he was disorganized and psychotic much of the time, I believed he was telling me that it was important to him to be someone with the dignity and capacity of a working person. I let him know that I respected this part of him but that in reality he stood a better chance of being employed if he were to receive financial assistance. This would permit him to attend to his health, be more mobile, and have a more socially acceptable physical appearance. I was also concerned about his health and safety and felt it was necessary to improve his situation before going further into psychodynamic issues. Medications were a moot point—he adamantly refused to take them.

It took close to a year for Mr. D. to sign an application for disability. In order to achieve this goal, I had to understand why he seemed to be so comfortable with his miserable personal hygiene and appearance and why he needed to repeat incessantly his catchphrase about finding work. He seemed to need my understanding of how important these symptoms were to his basic sense of existence before he could let down his resistance. He needed to know that I did not want to take anything away from him. I had to find a way, without offering interpretations (which were not well received), to reassure him that I wanted to give to him and not to take away. His years of playing the role of chronic mental patient had left him with little concern about how he appeared to others. Perhaps he understood but could not verbalize that the symptoms were important pieces of his identity. I was the one who was upset about the condition he was in, while he was relatively comfortable with his poor hygiene and marginality. It was as if he were saying to me that I would not be able to help him at all unless I finally understood how much he felt he had to lose if he were to change. As soon as I realized this, he did begin to change.

Mr. D.'s ritualistic verbalizations and behaviors were important parts of his presentation of self. There was a strange quality to the repetitions— they seemed to have an important purpose, yet I sensed their meaning should not be interpreted. Although the obsessive thoughts and compulsive behaviors were controlling him, they did not take the form of voices telling him what to do. Rather, they seemed to be actions that helped him maintain an inner sense of continuity. For instance, they were most noticeable when he entered or left a room, as if passing through an external boundary threatened his inner sense of boundedness, and the enhanced ritualistic behavior somehow helped him contain the resulting anxiety. Similarly, his verbalizations became repetitive and seemed to me somewhat ritualistic whenever he was made anxious by our discussions about ways in which he might need to change.

His obsessive thoughts and ritualistic behaviors were involved in the maintenance of his sense of identity in isolation from interpersonal relatedness, and the issue seemed to be his very existence. Thomas Ogden (1989) speaks of an "autistic-contiguous organization" of experience and explains the importance of this primitive system for maintaining an identity: "The autistic-contiguous organization is associated with a specific mode of attributing meaning to experience in which raw sensory data are ordered by means of forming pre-symbolic connections between sensory impressions that come to constitute bounded surfaces. Freud: 'The ego (the I) is first and foremost a bodily ego.' . . . In an autistic-contiguous mode, it is experiences of sensation, particularly at the skin surface, that are the principle media for the creation of psychological meaning and the rudiments of the experience of the self" (p. 6).

The obsessive, perseverating, ritualistic behaviors exhibited by Mr. D qualify as autistic-contiguous. Another equivalent physical expression of self is his need to have a distinctive exterior covered with layers of smelly clothing. In our work with chronic patients, we are easily put off by this kind of behavioral manifestation, including those individuals who seem hopelessly preoccupied with their weak or degenerating physical condition. The frustration we feel when we fail in our feeble attempts to translate the physical appearance into shared psychological meanings parallels the patient's own fatalistic fear of internal disorganization and incurable illness. When serious character pathology goes untreated for years, these conditions and symptoms become deeply entrenched. Chronic patients who are in poor health, shabbily attired, and isolated become attached to their condition and tend to feel that there is no other way for them to know themselves or to maintain an identity. Efforts to remove unpleasant symptoms may be doomed to failure unless the symptoms are understood and accepted as necessary expressions of a basic sense of self.

A few months after commencing therapy, Mr. D. moved into a board-and-care home. Before, he had been in hiding—blending into the urban landscape, unnoticeable among the other street people and chronically mentally ill—and was able to get away with his unkempt appearance. Now he was among more closely watched residents and was not permitted to build an exterior layer of rags and dirt. He was made to clean up and attend to personal hygiene. Soon thereafter, he developed a collection of new obsessive, ritualistic body movements and behaviors that seemed to take the place of the filthy and ragged exterior identity that had been taken away. For instance, he would need to retrace his steps in the hallway outside my office before entering and would carefully hold out his arms as if they were wings and he was carefully "landing" in his chair.

Meanwhile, Mr. D. began to engage me in an extended handshake routine at the beginning of each session. Any attempt to interpret such behavior proved futile. But my participation in the ritual, as well as my understanding that he needed to have some kind of physical contact with me, seemed to enable him to accept the kind of human contact that was so sorely lacking in his life. When my hand and arm movements fell into the correct rhythm and synchronized with his, our eyes met, and it was understood that we could now take our seats and proceed with an interaction in a verbal mode.

In slightly less than two years of once-a-week psychodynamic psychotherapy, Mr. D. has emerged from an isolated internal world of relative nonrelatedness. Living in a board-and-care home provides a certain amount of safety and social interaction. He no longer hides behind an encrusted, semiautistic layer of rags and filth. He comes to his therapy sessions regularly and engages with me somewhat spontaneously, without the endless rituals. Now there is a quality of human contact, with me and in his everyday life, that he says makes him feel like a human being once again.

Conclusion

Impasses occur at every stage of psychotherapy. At first, the patient is reluctant to begin therapy. When the therapist makes recommendations— such as my recommendations to Mr. D. that he move into a board-and-care home and apply for disability benefits—the client does not follow through. When there is a certain amount of improvement in the patient's condition, he or she becomes ambivalent about proceeding, and there may be missed appointments. In the public mental health clinic, especially when the patient suffers from a severe mental disorder and demonstrates a great deal of ambivalence about being in relationships, about dependency and growth, the impasses can be disconcerting for the therapist, eventually leading to frustration, burnout, and a feeling of failure.

It can be reassuring for the therapist to read accounts, in the literature of psychoanalysis and psychodynamic psychotherapy, of impasses just like the ones encountered in the public clinic. And the deeper meaning that analysts attribute to the impasse somehow reminds the clinician that they are expert practitioners and that something more important is going on here than a simple matter of a social servant offering a marginal citizen a service that the latter does not want. As clinicians in the public sector are able (when they have the time and interest) to immerse themselves in the psychodynamic formulations and therapeutic strategies that make up the professional literature and the continuing education curriculum of their specialties, they will find helpful tips for those moments of hair-pulling, as well as an intellectual challenge that makes some of the more routine and monotonous parts of their work bearable.

In light of the recent awareness of the plight of today's chronic patient, clinicians must recognize the need to treat the inner experience of chronicity in addition to providing assistance with the external problems and deficiencies. It may seem an impossible task to get through layers of hardened defensiveness and resistance. And it is much easier to fall back to the task of designing minimal treatment plans that are deemed more "realistic." But it often proves rewarding to attend to the psychodynamics of chronicity in the community mental health setting. As in the case of Mr. D., it may be possible to loosen a deeply entrenched defensiveness and reach the patient. He may never achieve a "cure" for the fundamental pathology, but important improvements can occur because of the clinician's efforts to understand. If we are to provide a truly humane treatment, we must help this group of patients transcend aspects of their entrenched presentation of self, and in doing so we must attend not only to their literal and concrete presentation and needs but also to what is symbolic and intrapsychic.

References

Bachrach, L. L., and Lamb, H. R. "What Have We Learned from Deinstitutionalization?" *Psychiatric Annals*, 1989, *19* (1), 12–21.

Goffman, E. *Asylums: Essays on the Social Situation of Mental Patients and Other Inmates.* New York: Anchor/Doubleday, 1961.

Kupers, T. A. "The 'Chronic' Problem." In T. A. Kupers, *Public Therapy: The Practice of Psychotherapy in the Public Mental Health Clinic.* New York: Free Press, 1981.

Lamb, H. R. *Treating the Long-Term Mentally Ill.* San Francisco: Jossey-Bass, 1982.

Lamb, H. R., and Zusman, J. "A New Look at Primary Prevention." *Hospital and Community Psychiatry*, 1981, *32*, 843–847.

Ogden, T. "On the Concept of an Autistic-Contiguous Position." *International Journal of Psychoanalysis*, 1989, *70*, 127–140.

Pepper, B., Kirshner, M., and Ryglewicz, H. "The Young Adult Chronic Patient: Overview of a Population." *Hospital and Community Psychiatry*, 1981, *32*, 463–469.

Scheff, T. *Being Mentally Ill: A Sociological Identity.* Hawthorne, N.Y.: Aldine, 1966.

Test, M. A., and Stein, L. I. "Community Treatment of the Chronic Patient: Research Overview." *Schizophrenia Bulletin*, 1978, *4*, 350–364.

Zusman, J. "Some Explanations of the Changing Appearance of Psychotic Patients." *Millbank Memorial Fund Quarterly*, 1966, *44*, 234–256.

Zusman, J., and Lamb, H. R. "In Defense of Community Mental Health." *American Journal of Psychiatry*, 1977, *134*, 887–890.

Richard Bloom is a staff psychologist in the outpatient department of Berkeley Mental Health Services and has a private practice in Berkeley, California.

Psychodynamic principles and a therapeutic community model are utilized in a halfway house for adults.

Community as Therapy

Elizabeth K. Gardner

I am the site director of Manzanita House, a psychiatric halfway house that operates as a transitional program for mentally disordered adults who are attempting to achieve some level of independent living, either after being discharged from a psychiatric hospital or after leaving their families. We are a small facility with fourteen beds and a staff of eight. Our program blends elements of a social rehabilitation model (Anthony and Liberman, 1986) and a therapeutic community model (Peck, 1987). The effectiveness of our program depends not only on educating our residents in basic living skills (such as hygiene, budgeting, and communication) but also on educating them in what it means to be an adult.

The last is what we consider to be our primary task. We help residents learn to take responsibility for themselves and to experience themselves as acting rather than merely being acted on in their lives. In the process of learning better hygiene, participating in individual counseling sessions, or chairing a business meeting, they have opportunities to learn to be adults. But practical education and training in living skills are not sufficient to accomplish the task.

Residents enter our program with the conscious desire to improve their independent living skills. At the same time that they consciously desire this, they also have unconscious desires—for instance, to be taken care of in the way they never were as children. In addition, they have developed a variety of defenses to help them cope in the world, some of which help them while others hurt them. When left unaddressed and unexamined, these unconscious desires and defenses can render a program impotent to effect change; it can even tear a program apart.

The staff also brings unconscious desires and defenses to their work,

New Directions for Mental Health Services, no. 46, Summer 1990 © Jossey-Bass Inc., Publishers and these must also be examined since they, too, have the ability to affect a program for better or worse. Parallel process has become an integral part of our work, and it has taught us the degree to which staff and residents are dynamically interrelated. For example, when residents are too dependent on staff, it is often the case that the residents are finding all-to-ready caretakers among the staff. Generally, this does not occur consciously. Staff do not consciously think, "Gee, since you would like me to fix you, I would be more than happy to do so." Instead, the staff become aware of this only after they have spent considerable time soul-searching as a group. And the impetus for staff self-examination might at first seem unrelated to conflicts about dependency. The process might begin with the staff airing feelings of being "burned out" or feelings of resentment toward residents.

The Value of the Therapeutic Community

Operating as a therapeutic community has provided our program with a powerful means of effecting change in the lives of our residents. Residents are given opportunities to be involved actively in the running of the community, and they are charged with responsibility for all that occurs in the community. Like staff, they are asked to participate in studying the problems and difficulties that occur and in arriving collectively at solutions. Jansen (1980) describes the therapeutic community as a setting in which all members are joined in the "fullest exploration of the issues," with the shared goal of getting help with their "psychological difficulties within a structure specifically designed to illuminate personal problems by involving people directly in community living and encouraging face-to-face encounters" (p. 24). Jansen developed the Richmond Fellowship in 1959, which includes a number of halfway houses all over the world. He considers it the aim of a therapeutic community to help its members eventually leave the community "in order to live as a viable member of society" (p. 24). The programs in the Richmond Fellowship all draw on psychoanalytic theory and technique in order to have a means of working with the unconscious dynamics and defenses that occur among the community members.

The Use of Psychodynamic Principles

Some of the unconscious undercurrents and dynamics that occur in our community are quite formidable, and if they are not interpreted, analyzed, and worked through, they have the potential to undermine residents' efforts to avoid chronicity. Regardless of their particular mental illness, residents tend to belie their verbal intent to accept more adult responsibility with behavior that exhibits resistance at every turn. Typically, they do this either by remaining lethargic and disinterested or by battling with staff over rules and program policies. Their behavior guarantees their status as "mental patients," despite their conscious stated intention to become less dependent or even to get out of the mental health system. It is only by addressing these behaviors psychodynamically that one is able to confront the unconscious conflicts that fuel them.

This process can be a pivotal piece of work. By making conscious the unconscious themes that the residents are acting out, the staff help the residents become more knowledgeable about themselves. Knowledge is power, and the mentally ill need as much power as they can get in order to mobilize their resources and achieve their goals. Making conscious does not mean simply confronting what is going on; it also means understanding what is going on and offering alternative strategies to attain what is desired.

The Example of Manzanita House

My belief in the value of using psychodynamic theory and techniques within a therapeutic community comes from my experience of seeing it actually transform a program that was about to be discontinued into a program that is successful. When I became site director at Manzanita House in 1988, the program was in disarray. The census for the program, as well as the average length of stay for residents, had been so poor in the past that the county was giving the program notice that it must improve or its funding would end. The residents were flagrantly rebelling against most aspects of the program, demanding loudly that staff make them better and then blaming them for their failure to do so. The staff were autocratically attempting to keep order in the house, just as loudly demanding that residents do their programs, and blaming them for their failure to do so. The staff were beleaguered and burned out, viewing themselves as under attack from all sides. When asked why things were such a mess, the staff typically responded by blaming the county, the parent organization, or the residents. Conversely, the residents responded by blaming either the staff or less familiar outside entities who they believed were making the lives of their staff miserable.

The program was being held together by the sheer force of will of the senior counselor who, after the previous director's abrupt departure, was running the program with a lot of heart and an iron fist. Her marine-with-a-heart approach evoked a great deal of affection and loyalty from the staff and residents, and it at least held them together in the face of all the problems. But despite her best efforts, the program was on the verge of collapse. Staff and residents were continuing to engage in enervating power struggles, and the census was continuing to drop. Residents' failure to do their programs was consistently viewed as their fault, and there was no examination of the way in which staff were working with the residents. Similarly, if a staff member was failing to do his or her job, it was considered to be strictly his or her fault. There was no self-reflection or examination of what other factors might be contributing to or determining these situations. As in the worst dysfunctional families, when staff or residents were not doing what they should be doing, they were blamed for their failures and became the identified patients. Blame, scapegoating, and arguing were the prevailing means of expressing conflict.

Coming into this community felt like entering the lion's den—it was terrifying and exciting at the same time. The senior counselor imbued the program with her passionate spirit, and the open and direct battles that sometimes occurred with staff were lively, to say the least. But nowhere did I feel safe. Luckily, the senior counselor quit shortly after I was hired. Then, to a degree with her blessing, I had the opportunity to do what I felt needed to be done in order to save the program. Her departure created an opportunity for change, and the staff were more than ready to try a new approach that might offer them relief from the battle, plus an opportunity to save their jobs.

Clearly the first step toward getting the house in order would be to address the acting out. My initial efforts to do so were largely unsuccessful. All of my clinical observations, interpretations, and interventions went for naught. The staff continued to "react to" rather than "work with" the residents and each other, without any awareness of their part in these ongoing dynamics. They persisted in remaining deeply entrenched in an "us-versus-them" mentality.

As I listened to them, I began to understand how such a bright and capable staff had gotten so stuck. I discovered that I was not the only one who felt unsafe. The "us-versus-them" mentality had helped them cope with a number of experiences in the past few years that had threatened their safety and undermined their trust. As a result, they were too afraid to reveal their true selves to one another, and without this, no one among them could be open to any actual change. The first order of business then was to create a model of working together that would enable staff to rebuild trust and feel safe enough to reveal more of themselves to each other. After participating in a Tavistock training (Rice, 1965) and reading Peck's (1987) view of community making, I determined that becoming a therapeutic community was the most compelling means of accomplishing this task.

Main (1980), who originally coined the term "therapeutic community," defines it as follows: "It involves the total community in a culture of inquiry into the nature of the social processes within" (p. 55). One of the hallmarks of a therapeutic community is that the responsibility for what is working and is not working is shared by *all* members of the community. It would no longer be acceptable to view Manzanita's failures as solely the fault of one or several individuals. Becoming a therapeutic community mandated reflection and group study of any and all problems. This kind of collective self-scrutiny also offered us a means of breaking the entrenched assumption of dependency (Bion, 1961)—namely, the collusion between staff and residents in avoiding anxiety related to conflict and programmatic change by depending on someone to take care of them. While the residents attempted to be dependent on the staff, the staff in turn depended on the senior counselor. The senior counselor's autocratic approach to running the program tended to encourage this behavior, since it infantilized the residents as well as the staff. Whatever residents and staff could not or would not do, she would do for them. Her resentment toward residents and staff was equaled only by the resentment that staff felt toward residents and residents toward staff. My initial interventions in helping us to become a therapeutic community were aimed at ending this kind of pseudodependency.

Main (1980) writes that the aim of a therapeutic community is to create "together a social system based not on a medical model of a healthy knowledgeable staff and sick obedient patients, but on the joint recognition of each individual's capacity and limitations for performing essential tasks, and with participation by all in arranging that these be carried out" (p. 53). This type of social system would make it difficult for staff or anyone at Manzanita to maintain an "us-versus-them" mentality. Blame and scapegoating cannot thrive in such an environment.

Peck (1987) defines the development of community in terms of four stages: pseudocommunity, chaos, emptiness, and community. When we began the process of becoming a therapeutic community, we were somewhere between the first two stages. The staff would start to get into conflicts with each other and then would quickly retreat to the comfort of acting as if there were no conflicts. The pull toward remaining a "pseudocommunity" was strong, since it offered at least the safety of superficial closeness. An understanding of Peck's views on community making, however, encouraged the staff to believe that if we could tolerate the chaos of trying to convert and control each other and then intentionally empty ourselves of the need to do these things (in other words, if we could truly open ourselves to each other), then we could become a real community. We decided that we first had to experience this openness as a staff if we were to help the residents and ourselves become a therapeutic community. But the realities of parallel process made this less of a sequential process than we had anticipated because, as we were changed as a staff, so in turn were the residents, and so in turn was our program.

The staff took on the challenge of moving through Peck's stages by meeting twice a month for two hours of unstructured, leaderless process. All of us were charged with the specific task of bringing to or discovering in these meetings what was blocking us from accepting each other and then of finding ways either to work through these blocks or to set them aside. All of us retained the right to refuse to say or do anything that we did not, for whatever reason, feel comfortable saying or doing. All of us had read Peck's "stages of community making" and Bion's (1961) theory of group dynamics, so we knew basically what we were going to be up against and what we needed to do to get through it. Our meetings began much like Quaker meetings, with silence and contemplation, until someone felt the desire to speak. This procedure developed in response to Peck's suggestion that silence and contemplation could be invaluable tools in becoming a community.

In adopting Bion's theory, we were adopting the belief that parallel process is omnipresent in groups. In other words, one's individual identity is at times subsumed by the group. When speaking at any given moment, a group member may be functioning as a spokesperson for the group as well as for himself or herself. Adopting this theory forced us as a staff to listen differently to each other. It was not possible to react so quickly to one another since it was not possible to know, without reflection, to whom or what we were reacting. Initially, staff continued the habit of trying to blame and scapegoat each other. This began to change as the staff shared their feelings for each other and learned more about the types of defenses that group members or groups use to ward off their anxieties.

By meeting together, the staff learned when their behavior was defensive. For instance, they began to see that sometimes when they thought they were confronting one another in an appropriate way, they were actually scapegoating or blaming. The more these defenses became conscious and recognizable, the more we as a staff were able to risk sharing our true selves with each other. As Peck predicted, we became increasingly able to share our "brokenness" (our fears, insecurities, and so on) with each other. Peck maintains that "it is only among the overtly imperfect that we can find community" (p. 231). Prior to engaging in these process meetings, the staff had made every effort to protect and preserve their images of themselves as overtly perfect staff members. The frequent usage of blame had evoked a counterdefensive posture of blamelessness. When a staff member had been accused of doing something wrong, the exchange had typically boiled down to "I did not!" "You did, too!" Or there had been silent acquiescence to the tirade of blame.

Initially, it was easier for me to spot the individual and group defenses when they were happening because I was not lost in the forest, and I had more formal training in group dynamics. So I often took the lead in commenting on and educating staff about these behaviors when they occurred. But as time went on and staff became more conscious of group dynamics and were able to trust each other more, I was able to pull back and they were able to take on more of the process work. I was also able to risk getting lost in the forest with them and depending on them, not just me, to get us out. Becoming a community means that every member takes on a leadership role, and Peck contends that for this to happen the designated leader of the group has to be willing to fall from grace in the group's eyes as the omniscient, omnipotent one. It was not until I was able to admit to the staff that I did not know everything and could not do everything for them (in Peck's terms, to die as the group leader) that staff were able to embrace their leadership responsibilities as members of the group.

Meanwhile, of course, the whole community was changing. As staff became willing to drop their guard with each other and to assume more responsibility for themselves, they were able to facilitate the residents' doing the same. The locus of treatment began to shift from the individual sessions that staff had with residents to the formal and informal group meetings; in other words, the program was shifting from an outpatient model of treatment to a therapeutic community model. Staff were tending to blame residents less for not doing their programs and, instead, to be curious about what was not working and to explore these difficulties with the community as a whole. The "us-versus-them" model of relating between staff and residents began to fall away, and residents began taking more risks and encountering each others' differences, just as staff were doing. As I had done with staff, so staff in turn did with residents. Initially, they assumed active leadership in helping residents become conscious of when they were confronting each other in inappropriate or defensive ways and when they were actually meeting each other. As the residents became more educated and adept at recognizing these defenses, staff pulled back and allowed them to take more of the lead in the process work.

Gradually, we became a therapeutic community. Problem behaviors were designated as the responsibility of *every* member of the community. Residents and staff began working together to remedy these situations. One of our first formal program changes was the addition of impromptu house meetings to our milieu work. We decided that any of us (staff or residents) could call a house meeting any time we felt the need for community support or assistance. A number of experiences using impromptu house meetings to address problems made clear to us the power of house meetings in helping a new resident weather the initial adjustment period. For example, one new resident, "Bill," was having a hard time bonding with the program. He was terrified of staying, and after only a few days he became agitated, withdrawn, and anxious to leave. One morning, he was pacing throughout the house and announced to me and another staff person (Larry) that he was leaving. Despite private meetings with Larry and me in which we attempted to clarify what was troubling him, to offer him support, and to suggest ways of coping with his anxieties, Bill remained tense, agitated, and determined to leave. On an impulse, I decided to call a house meeting to help Bill decide what he wanted to do. This was a risky intervention since Bill was an extremely shy and guarded young man who communicated minimally and often inaudibly with others. Ignoring these concerns, Larry and I gathered the residents together in the recreation room along with Bill and explained to them that Bill was feeling scared and wanted to leave the program. With little encouragement from us, the residents started asking Bill what he was afraid of, and with remarkable ease, Bill started sharing his feelings with them, more even than he had shared with either of us. By the end of the exchange, Bill decided that he wanted to stay.

Prior to becoming a therapeutic community, this situation would have been considered solely the province of the staff, and they would have responded accordingly. The residents would have expected staff to fix Bill, and the staff would have done their best to do so. Clearly this type of intervention would not have worked. Larry and I had done our best, but it was the community intervention that made the difference.

The outcome of instituting these changes at Manzanita House has been good. From the outset, I had made it clear to our parent organization and the county that we were going to be in chaos for a while longer before we got better, and I asked them to leave us alone and not pass judgment on the success of our venture for at least six months. By the middle of my first year, we were honored for program excellence by our parent organization, and we were off probation. By the end of the year, we were able to meet our county contract (by maintaining the necessary census) for the first time in years.

Conclusion

Halfway houses have tended to eschew psychodynamic theories and techniques in favor of a social rehabilitation model of treatment, largely in an effort to prevent the dehumanizing and pathologizing aspects of the medical model (Main, 1980; Szasz, 1961; Laing, 1965) from thwarting or undermining mentally ill adults in their efforts to achieve their goals. The therapeutic community model was developed to correct these aspects of the medical model. By creating "an atmosphere of respect for all difficulties" we move "a long way from the medical model, whereby disease is skillfully treated in anonymous people under a blanket medical compassion and served by a clinically aloof and separate administration" (Main, 1977, p. 3, cited in Kennard, 1983, p. 46). Our model of a therapeutic community borrows from Main, Bion (1961), Jones (1953), and especially from Peck (1987), who goes even further in humanizing the medical model with his deeply spiritual and disciplined perspective. By using this model, we were able to transform ourselves from a "pseudo-community" into a community in which psychodynamic theories and techniques can be used by the community and the individuals involved to effect change in the lives of mentally ill adults.

References

Anthony, W. A., and Liberman, R. P. "The Practice of Psychiatric Rehabilitation: Historical, Conceptual, and Research Base." *Schizophrenia Bulletin,* 1986, *12* (4), 542–559.

Bion, W. R. *Experiences in Groups.* New York: Basic Books, 1961.

Jansen, E. (ed.). *The Therapeutic Community.* London: Croom Helm, 1980.

Jones, M. *The Therapeutic Community: A New Treatment Method in Psychiatry.* New York: Basic Books, 1953.

Kennard, D. *An Introduction to Therapeutic Communities.* London: Routledge & Kegan Paul, 1983.

Laing, R. D. *The Divided Self.* New York: Penguin Books, 1965.

Main, T. "The Concept of the Therapeutic Community: Variations and Vicissitudes." *Group Analysis,* 1977, *10* (2), supplement 1–24.

Main, T. "Some Basic Concepts in Therapeutic Community Work." In E. Jansen (ed.), *The Therapeutic Community.* London: Croom Helm, 1980.

Peck, M. S. *The Different Drum.* New York: Simon & Schuster, 1987.

Rice, A. K. *Learning for Leadership.* London: Tavistock Publications, 1965.

Szasz, T. F. *The Myth of Mental Illness.* New York: Hoedner-Harper, 1961.

Elizabeth K. Gardner is site director of Manzanita House, Union City, California.

Understanding the plight of homeless persons within the context of catastrophic events leads to a multifocal treatment strategy.

Reflections on Working with the Homeless

Christine A. Seeger

The faces of the poor in the United States without a place to call home are different today than they were a generation ago (Stark, 1987). We are now faced with a rapidly growing heterogeneous homeless population of men, women, children (San Francisco Board of Supervisors' Task Force, 1989), adolescents, the elderly, the disabled, and families. Counting those without homes is difficult. Wright and Weber (1987) estimate the homeless population nationwide to vary from 350,000 to 3 or 4 million. Estimates regarding the prevalence of mental illness, substance abuse, and medical illness among the homeless also vary widely (Snow, Baker, Anderson, and Martin, 1986; Bassuk, 1984; Bean, Stelf, and Howe, 1987; Surber, Pwyer, Goldfinger, and Kelly, 1988). The homeless are subject to extreme poverty, high levels of disability, and social isolation (Rossi, Wright, Fisher, and Willis, 1987). Due to circumstances beyond their immediate control, they are unable to acquire and maintain permanent housing. As a result, they must live in city streets, subways, parks, public shelters, abandoned cars or buildings, or, when lucky, in crowded and sometimes dangerous single room occupancy hotels (SROs).

I am mental health director of the San Francisco Health Care for the Homeless Project, which is one of nineteen pilot projects across the nation originally funded by the Robert Wood Johnson Foundation. Our mandate was to provide medical and mental health services to this underserved population. We designed a multidisciplinary team consisting of mental health workers, social workers, nurse practitioners, and outreach workers. We have held clinics in public shelters and drop-in centers serving the homeless, and we have spent many long hours on the streets developing therapeutic relationships.

In this chapter, I will briefly outline the multifocal treatment strategy we have developed (Blackwell and others, in press). Our work is informed by an understanding of homelessness as a stressor comparable to catastrophic events such as earthquake and war, and I will next describe this formulation and mention ways in which it informs our therapeutic practice. Finally, we have discovered that, in order to be effective with homeless clients, we mental health providers must gain their trust by demonstrating not only an understanding of their plight but also a willingness to leave our offices and join them in their attempts to improve their situation. I will end with some examples of ways in which staff can collaborate with homeless clients.

A Multifocal Treatment Strategy

In our work with homeless people, the goal is always the establishment of a permanent, stable housing situation and integration into a community that meets the client's needs for support. We have found that the most effective strategy uses a combination of social advocacy and psychodynamic principles.

Social advocacy involves a willingness on the part of the "therapist" to become involved in the client's acquisition of such things as financial entitlements, housing, medical services, legal assistance, community support services, childcare, and so on. This may include making referrals, advocating with an agency to serve the client, escorting the client to appointments, or using any other appropriate means of ensuring improvement in the client's material circumstances. Despite the obvious practical implications of such strategies, this assistance begins to create small experiences of success and begins to rebuild the client's trust in his or her capacity to effect change. It also strengthens the image of the therapist as an effective, caring, trustworthy assistant.

The psychological strategy has three aspects: validating the client's feeling that circumstances are overwhelming; clarifying that he or she must take an active, responsible role in improving the situation; and providing support and treatment for concomitant problems such as substance abuse, diagnosable mental or medical problems, or underlying grief or anger about being homeless. Obviously, the psychological strategy and the therapist's role as social advocate are interconnected. One strengthens the other.

An important principle to keep in mind is that homeless people are frequently ignored, insulted, or humiliated on the streets. A caring, respectful approach and a willingness to listen are powerful invitations to communication. One of our outreach workers mentioned that he felt every interaction he had on the street was a form of therapy because he affirmed each person's dignity and showed acceptance of that person's right to be who and where he or she was.

Since we are talking about a group of people with a damaged sense of trust, it is particularly important to involve each individual in his or her own needs assessment. Some people may enumerate food, clothing, or shelter as a present need, but there are others who request only such things as a pair of sunglasses, a sleeping bag, or clean socks. It may take time to develop a relationship before further services can be provided. There are other folks for whom treatment of a medical or psychiatric disorder must be rendered before proceeding. Each individual must be recognized, their story told and listened to, and their pace of change respected.

Leah is a sixty-six-year-old single woman I met in a women's shelter where she had been living for approximately four months. She came to the women's discussion group we were holding once a week at the shelter in the evening at the time the women were allowed in for the night. She was always clean in appearance and hygiene. She carried her belongings in several large bags, as did the other women, since they had to be out of the shelter during the day. She kept herself isolated and did not appear to have any friends, although she was friendly to several other women. She came to the group fairly regularly. She was quiet and would reveal little personal information, but she seemed to develop a warm relationship with us. Over the ensuing months, she refused to follow up on any suggestions about applying for Social Security, a refusal that revealed clues to what later was discovered to be a fixed delusion. It took close to a year to piece together her story. She believed that Ronald Reagan, while governor of California, had made a deal with her to give her funds for the mentally ill and that he had not followed through. In the process she believed her identification and her identity had been stolen, and her seventeen-year-old son had been killed or kidnapped. She had been traveling around the country on buses for the past twenty years looking for this son. She had supported herself for a time doing menial jobs until she had injured her leg on a job. She had relied on handouts and social services since then.

We met with her weekly in the group and privately. She enjoyed talking with us as long as we didn't probe too deeply into her life. We began to introduce the idea of a nearby safe hotel in which we worked. We made arrangements with the social support staff in the hotel to accept her without money and to help her apply for welfare after entry. We accompanied her to her intake appointment. When she was accepted, she was very reluctant to go. We supported her moving into the room but identified times she could return to the shelter and visit. We helped her move and visited her regularly with one of the shelter staff. We encouraged her hobbies of reading and sewing, including bringing her a used sewing machine for Christmas.

She has steadfastly refused to apply for Social Security or to receive psychiatric services at the mental health clinic. She will at times talk about her fears when they begin to interfere with her daily activities and sleeping. She remains isolated but is independent, safely housed, receives financial benefits, and is living within a small community of caregivers.

Leah was sheltered when we met her, but her life-style was a hardship. She was required to spend her days outside during all kinds of weather, regardless of her age and braced leg. She had no privacy, few choices, and no place to call her own. On first appearance her psychotic disorder was well hidden, but it prevented her from improving her situation. We never confronted her beliefs regarding Social Security, and we confirmed that the world can be dangerous without protection. At the same time, we befriended her and introduced her to a shelter social worker whom she grew to trust. We then were able to find a living situation that conformed to her particular needs and to offer it as protection and safety. We allowed her to pace herself slowly and offered change with personal support.

Homelessness and Other Catastrophes

Our ability to provide services rests on an ability to understand homelessness. I find it useful to consider the phenomenon in this country in relation to other catastrophic events, such as earthquakes, floods, and war. By doing so, we put the problem and its effects in a perspective that permits us to make use of a certain amount of research on catastrophic events, and then we are better able to assess accurately the level and kind of response that is needed.

In natural disasters and war, a large number of people experience the personal loss of home, possessions, job, community, and the structuring of time and purpose that these things usually provide. The trauma has profound and lasting effects on the routines, experiences, and quality of everyday life. Coles (1989) discusses the psychological consequences of being without a home and describes the homeless children he interviewed as "transients or wanderers in the mind." He believes the children are describing not only literal homelessness but also an experience of being at loose ends and estranged from fellow human beings.

Torres (1989), who directed a mental health program in one of New York's largest men's shelters in the Bronx, compares the sheltered men to the refugee population he worked with in Nicaragua. According to Torres, the men in the shelter showed more depression, apathy, and evidence of psychological dysfunction. He believes this was due to the lack of a unifying purpose or understandable cause to explain the loss of home and social fabric among the residents of the shelter.

Our observations match those of Torres. Consider the case of Mr. P., a forty-two-year-old married man I met in a men's shelter. He had been homeless with his wife and two children for six months since the factory he had worked in had closed. They had left their community in search of work, which he had been unable to find. They did not want to be a burden on their family and friends back home, but they missed the sense of belonging they had with them. Mr. P. was then separated from his wife and children because of arguments and discord resulting from his unemployment and their inability to reestablish a home. He felt despondent and uncertain about whether he could put his life back together. Beyond that, he felt he really did not know what had gone wrong, what had caused the downward spiral, and because he could not find any other cause, he had only himself to blame for his unfortunate predicament. Self-blame was an obvious feature of his depression.

Cohen and Ahearn (1980), in their work with flood and earthquake victims, and Erikson (1976), in his study of Buffalo Creek survivors, discuss the psychological importance of loss of one's social fabric. Erikson describes "a blow to the tissues of social life that damages the bonds linking people together. The collective trauma works its way slowly and even insidiously into the awareness of those who suffer from it . . . [leading to] a gradual realization that the community no longer exists as a source of nurturance and that a part of the self has disappeared" (p. 302).

By definition, homelessness implies the lack of a supportive social network that would have prevented the homeless condition. This means that family or friends are not available as resources to provide physical and emotional shelter and that the homeless individual or family is in a state of material poverty, unable to secure a safe, comfortable living arrangement. It is frequently a combination of factors—lack of affordable housing, difficulty in finding work, or inability to compete in the job market in addition to mental, emotional, or physical disability—that leads individuals to the dead-end circumstance of homelessness. The process of becoming homeless may be sudden, as when someone flees an abusive situation, but is more often an unfolding phenomenon in which an individual's social fabric is torn thread by thread, and he or she is not able to make the necessary repairs before another thread is broken. The process can be initiated by a plant closure, a job firing, an eviction, illness, accident, or loss of a supporting partner. For many, this can lead to an inability to make enough money to maintain or reestablish a housing situation, and then, in circular fashion, lack of housing severely handicaps the process of job acquisition. Family and friends may be called on initially for support, but this can create a tremendous strain on meager resources and on relationships. There are often time limits placed on this support and when this system is no longer viable, the individual or family is left with the difficult choice between moving to the streets or navigating through the highly complex bureaucracy of our social service system. All of this is made much more complicated by any untreated chemical dependency or emotional problem.

Homelessness has profound emotional and cognitive consequences. From our experience on the project, these consequences differ according to the length of time an individual has been homeless. The newly homeless show the effects (such as shock, confusion, and fear) of recently suffering a major devastating loss, but they are more likely to trust their capacity to reverse their situation. Those who have been homeless for months to years frequently have found adaptive mechanisms that allow them to tolerate their situation, and these mechanisms can interfere with their ability to make changes. This phenomenon appears to be described best by Seligman's (1975) concept of learned helplessness. Working in a laboratory setting, he studied animal and human subjects' response to a situation in which their best efforts did not avert negative outcome. He found that in a short period of time there was a decrease in the subject's motivation to try and affect the outcome, an interference in the process of learning new strategies to control the outcome, and if the unavoidable outcome was traumatic, the production of fear and depression. With the chronically homeless, we often find that initially they tried many strategies to improve their situation but to no avail. The long-term results are too often as Seligman outlines.

Kozol (1988), in his book *Rachel and Her Children,* stresses the uniformity of the mode of suffering of the homeless in New York, which he believes becomes institutionalized by their circumstances and by society's response. Similarly, Lifton and Olson (1976), in their analysis of the Buffalo Creek flood, state, "Without denying the existence of significant variation in psychological vulnerability, we have been far more impressed by the degree to which the massive character of the trauma subsumed individual differences and produced strikingly consistent forms of impairment" (p. 15).

Our experience leads us to agree with Kozol's observation that the stress inherent in the condition of homelessness makes the well sick and the unwell sicker. Consider the plight of Mrs. B., a forty-seven-year-old woman I met in a women's shelter. She had recently come to San Francisco with her four-year-old daughter after fleeing her alcoholic, abusive second husband. She had no money or personal items. She felt frightened, depressed, anxious, and overwhelmed. She believed herself to be unable to tend to her child's needs, but feared loss of custody. She required community residential mental health treatment to recover from her depression, but over time she was able to reestablish a home for her daughter and herself. Homelessness was clearly a major stressor and aggravated her depression.

Cohen and Ahearn (1980) found that psychological impairment correlates with the type and duration of the disaster; the degree of loss; the victims' role, coping skills, and support system; and the survivors' perception and interpretation of the catastrophe. Lifton and Olson (1976) explore the importance of the survivor finding meaning in the experience of the disaster. They found the process of recovery impeded when there was a combination of abuse, resentment, and dependency—unfortunately, a widespread combination of feelings and circumstances for the homeless. They found the necessary conditions for improvement of the victims' mental health to be recognition of their suffering, acknowledgment of the causes of the disaster, the opportunity to rebuild their lives, and a general sense that the moral world had been righted again. We have found a similar combination of conditions necessary for reintegration of chronically homeless persons back into a community.

Social Action

Lifton and Olson (1976) define the concept of "survivor mission" as the taking of wisdom gleaned from a traumatic experience and putting it to a positive use. They found important positive psychological consequences in the capacity of people to embark on a collective mission that might contribute to the relief of others in similar situations. I believe that the grass-roots organizing of homeless people is just such a survivor mission and does have positive psychological consequences. In other words, when mental health staff join homeless clients in efforts to improve their situation, they not only build trust among the homeless that is necessary if they are to be effective providers but they also help homeless clients accomplish a survivor mission.

Andrew Hayes, a social worker on our project, is guided in his attempts to use community organizing as a supplemental mental health treatment by educator Paulo Freire's (1970) ideas about developing among disenfranchised people a more positive and potent sense of self, establishing a critical comprehension of the web of social reality, and cultivating resources and strategies for the attainment of personal and collective sociopolitical goals. Groups of homeless people who take political action and win improvements in social services do report that their successes make them feel more in control of their lives. Recently there was a large encampment of homeless people in a small park in front of San Francisco City Hall. Over time, this gathering of people living in tents became a focus of political tension among the homeless, the local government officials, and the police. As the situation developed, outreach workers and other health professionals from our project and from other agencies began developing relationships and providing services to those camped in the park. As tension heightened, several workers erected a tent in the park that was manned twenty-four hours a day. This allowed them better access to provide services as well as to stand in solidarity with the homeless. This also gave the workers a uniquely intimate relationship with the homeless community, fostering the development of trust and placing them in an important position to participate in the organizing of this community, to help stimulate indigenous leadership, and to help define the issues. In the end, the homeless were moved out of the park, but they were given access to free storage of their belongings for a month and offered prioritized access to social, mental health, and medical services. Perhaps most important, a number of people who participated in the community organizing have remained together and are planning a trip to Washington to participate in a national march and demonstration against homelessness. It will take time to evaluate the long-range effects of this activity, but many stated that for the first time in a long time they have some hope they can have an effect on their circumstances.

I will end with a quote from Anello (1989), our codirector of social work: "While there can be no doubt that the conditions of living experienced by the homeless have destructive and demoralizing impact or that many of the persons who have become homeless had preexisting social, psychological, and behavioral difficulties, the far more serious implication is that by failure to give social meaning to homelessness we permit the discarding of human beings who do have potential, who do have dreams and hopes, and who do have the capacity to succeed" (p. 2).

References

Anello, E. R. "A Social Welfare Approach to Homeless Women with Psychiatric Disorders." Unpublished manuscript, School of Social Welfare, University of California, Berkeley, 1989.

Bassuk, E. L. "The Homeless Problem." *Scientific American*, 1984, *251* (1), 40–45.

Bean, G. J., Jr., Stelf, M. E., and Howe, S. R. "Mental Health and Homelessness: Issues and Findings." *Social Work*, 1987, *32* (5), 411–416.

Blackwell, B., Breakey, W., Hammersley, D., Hammond, R., McMurray-Avila, M., and Seeger, C. A. "Psychiatric and Mental Health Services." In P. Brickner, L. Scharer, B. Conanan, and M. Savarese (eds.), *The Homeless and Healthcare: A Nationwide Experiment.* New York: Norton, in press.

Cohen, R. E., and Ahearn, F. L., Jr. *Handbook for Mental Health Care of Disaster Victims.* Baltimore: Johns Hopkins University Press, 1980.

Coles, R. "Lost Youth." *Vogue*, July 1989, pp. 186–189.

Erikson, K. T. "Loss of Communality at Buffalo Creek." *American Journal of Psychiatry*, 1976, *133* (3), 302–305.

Freire, P. *Pedagogy of the Oppressed.* New York: Seabury Press, 1970.

Kozol, J. *Rachel and Her Children.* New York: Fawcett Columbine Books, 1988.

Lifton, R. J., and Olson, E. "The Human Meaning of Total Disaster: The Buffalo Creek Experience." *Psychiatry*, 1976, *39*, 1–18.

Rossi, P., Wright, J., Fisher, G., and Willis, G. "The Urban Homeless: Estimating Composition and Size." *Science*, 1987, *235*, 1335–1341.

San Francisco Board of Supervisors' Task Force on Homeless Women and Children. "Homeless Women and Children in San Francisco." San Francisco: Board of Supervisors, 1989.

Seligman, M. *Helplessness: On Depression, Development and Death.* New York: W. H. Freeman, 1975.

Snow, D., Baker, S., Anderson, L., and Martin, M. "The Myth of Pervasive Mental Illness Among the Homeless." *Social Problems*, 1986, *33* (5), 407–423.

Stark, L. "From 'Winos' to 'Crazies': Demographics and Stereotypes of the Homeless." Unpublished manuscript, San Francisco, 1987.

Surber, R. W., Pwyer, K. J., Goldfinger, S. M., and Kelly, J. T. "Medical and Psychiatric Needs of the Homeless: A Preliminary Response." *Social Work*, 1988, *33* (2), 116–119.

Wright, J., and Weber, E. *Homelessness and Health.* Washington, D.C.: McGraw-Hill's Healthcare Information Center, 1987.

Christine A. Seeger is the mental health director and staff psychiatrist of the San Francisco Health Care for the Homeless Project. She is also the psychiatric consultant to the mental health crisis house, La Posada.

As client-consumer groups grow, their role in the design and implementation of community mental health services is enlarged. Just as the psychotherapist must pay attention to the client's desires, so must mental health providers pay close attention to the wishes of client-consumers and their potential contribution to the evolution of the service delivery system.

Collaboration Between Providers and Client-Consumers in Public Mental Health Programs

Ernest L. Silva

There has been a dramatic shift in the services provided by public mental health systems during the last twenty years. Not only has the trend been to move away from hospital-based services toward community-based services for those with ongoing severe mental disability but there has also been a concurrent shift in roles for the mentally disabled client, or consumer. Client-consumers are becoming actively involved as board members of agencies, as key program and administrative staff, as program developers, and as participants in service delivery systems. They are involved in the allocation of resources, the design of programs, the monitoring of service quality, and even in the provision of services in some programs. In other words, client-driven programs are rapidly evolving in many regions.

In some systems, providers view the change in clients' roles as an opportunity for creative collaboration between providers and consumers. In other locales, the response of providers to clients' demands for a larger role has been less enthusiastic, even defensive. Perhaps the clients' new level of participation is viewed as a threat to providers' already tenuous sense that they have some control over their working conditions. Since this shift in roles is a relatively recent development, it is not yet known what providers' response will be in many other systems. If administrators, clinicians at hospital and outpatient facilities, and staff of community support programs see the enlarged role for clients as an opportunity to improve the mental health delivery system and even to design a new role for themselves, then they will support the collaborative venture. If, on the other hand, the providers, already reeling from a relative diminution in their status, earning power, and job security brought on by the past decade's cuts in mental health budgets, view clients' strengthened position as a further encroachment on their own prerogatives, then they will resist the trend toward client-driven mental health programs.

Of course, the providers are not the only ones who can drag their feet. Clients can remain too unorganized to play a part. They sometimes have too great expectations and become visibly disappointed when projects move too slowly or result in too little change. They might choose to argue when effective collaboration would require that they compromise. And in individual cases, some of the difficulties they routinely have getting along with others may interfere with the collaborative process or the smooth running of programs. This is not to say that the clients' personal problems are primarily responsible for breakdowns in negotiations or that the clients will necessarily be the more unreasonable party in negotiations. But one of the main goals of this kind of collaboration is to help clients learn skills of social engagement. Sometimes therapists' most important contributions to this kind of collaboration are the talks they have on the sidelines with clients—for instance, when a therapist helps a client question his feelings that the person who argued against his proposal in a meeting was not out to get him, but rather to see the different perspectives brought into a program development process by different personalities. In other words, the psychotherapist's experience and expertise are often precisely what is needed to further the process of collaboration between consumers and providers, just as the therapist facilitates more effective collaboration between partners in a troubled marriage. Just as in a troubled marriage, however, it is rare that one partner is entirely at fault for the discord. In this chapter, I will not focus on therapists' sideline mini-interventions, nor will I focus on the clients' difficulties in joining in the collaboration. Rather, since my experience has been as an administrator and consultant to programs, I will focus on the providers' perspective.

Some consumer groups, agreeing with many professionals, have expressed the view that psychotherapy is not very effective in treating the severely mentally disabled and that psychopharmacology and social rehabilitation programs should be emphasized. Does this mean that when client-consumers are given more say in determining the shape of new programs, psychotherapists will be phased out of their jobs? Or as the collaboration evolves, will there be sufficient opportunity for psychotherapists, other providers and consumers to develop mutual trust, for the rigid polarization (psychotherapy versus social rehabilitation) to break down, and for all parties to see that there is a role for the therapist as well as the client in a modern comprehensive mental health system that includes inpatient and outpatient clinical programs, psychopharmacology, social rehabilitation programs, and client-driven programs?

I have been working in public mental health since 1969 and have been involved in the development of mental health programs ranging from acute care in a medical setting to client-driven services in the community. I have served as a manager in a public mental health system, an executive director of a community agency, and as consultant to county mental health divisions as well as to contract agencies. In each endeavor I have attempted to understand the political forces at play, including the power of united groups of client-consumers in the community, and I have attempted to help administrators, clinical staff, and client groups collaborate in the establishment of smooth-functioning service programs. A background in psychodynamic psychotherapy has helped in important ways. In the sections that follow, I will mention a few of the issues that regularly arise and suggest ways in which providers can help to make the transition to more collaborative efforts successful. Because of the confidential nature of some of the consultative work I have done and because the programs described are still in the early stages of development, I will not describe any particular project or organization by name. Rather, I will present anecdotes to illustrate issues. Before I do that, I will briefly review the background of client involvement in public mental health programs.

Evolution of a New Client Role

In the seventies, driven by rage about unreasonable constraint and mistreatment in psychiatric hospitals, outspoken client groups attacked the mental health system. They brought attention to intolerable state hospital conditions, the violation of patients' civil and legal rights, and the abuse of electroconvulsive therapy. As the number of vocal clients grew, so did the diversity of their areas of criticism. A political force developed that was focused on the deficits of the existing system (Brown, 1981). Unfortunately, these early efforts were easily dismissed. After cleaning up the worst abuses, providers were excused because they were seen by the public as "well intentioned," and the mentally disabled protesters were felt to be "unable to cope with realistic boundaries." Still, as the size and diversity of the client groups grew, their interests broadened, and some mental health providers began to see ways in which consumers of mental health services could play a valuable role in the provision of those services (Bloom and Asher, 1982). In some quarters, the client was beginning to be seen as a resource.

As client groups continued to evolve, they exhibited increased political savvy and power and more sophisticated organizational skills. Clients began providing self-help groups and demanding the right to participate in planning the allocation of limited mental health resources. In California, the Mental Health Services Reform Act of 1986 began a new phase of collaboration between consumers and providers and defined a new relationship between the mental health client and the mental health system. Clients had participated in the development of this act, and it clearly reflected a different orientation. Federal legislation, such as Public Law 99-660, already required an advisory role for consumers, but prior to 1986, in California at least, consumers' participation had been little more than token. Now there would be an opening for clients to define for themselves what their needs were, and they were to have real input into the design of programs to satisfy those needs. One of the first concrete changes was that mental health funds would be utilized to help clients find a place to live, and those clients would no longer need to undergo a psychiatric examination and be assigned a diagnosis in order to qualify for that help. This legislative change helped pave the way for client-driven mental health services. The clients had participated in developing a good product. In the process, they had seen that they could exert power and change the system.

How Are Providers to Manage in a Client-Driven Environment?

Effective staff participation in the design and implementation of a client-driven program requires of clinicians the same type of sensitivity, attention to dynamics, and innovative strategizing that are required if the psychotherapeutic relationship is to be successful (Kupers, 1981). Often I find that the greater the clinical skills of program designers and administrators, the greater the program's potential for success. Just as the psychotherapist attempts to foster the client's self-definition and initiative instead of prescribing a way for the client to behave in the consulting room, so the provider should attempt to maximize clients' participation in the design and operation of services.

There are ways for those who are sincere about the evolution of truly consumer-driven programs to transcend the resistance of service providers. For instance, providers who support enlarged client-consumer participation might pause to listen to the concerns of their less supportive colleagues and spend some time attending to those concerns. And planners who would like to guarantee real consumer participation might build safeguards into contracts between counties and the private, non-profit agencies that claim they want to establish client-driven programs. There might be a clause in the contract stating that if a program does not evolve into one where clients play an important role by a specified time limit, the parent agency will lose the contract for that program. This requirement is made instead of or in addition to the more familiar stipulation that the program's success will be measured by its record in meeting a specified schedule for start-up and full operation. The parent agency is left with a built-in motive to develop an autonomous, client-driven program.

It is sometimes not the strategy of advocates of client-driven programs within the mental health system that matters most. Rather, it is the moves made by the clients and the actual playing out of political events. For instance, in a community where a new public mental health service had been fully funded, one of a number of bidding agencies was selected to provide the service under contract to the local mental health department, and a start-up schedule was prepared for implementation. But there had been little, if any, canvassing of clients as to the selection of a provider before the contract was awarded to that agency.

A group of clients then met together and determined that they did not really want the agency that had been selected to run the program because they found that agency's philosophical orientation, track record of ignoring consumer input, and top-down administrative style objectionable. The client group was concerned that the agency would not be responsive to input from consumers of its services. The clients set out to obstruct the implementation of the program until their concerns were adequately addressed. In this case, the client group was very successful in organizing community support for their stand, and their efforts resulted in a change in the agency selected to provide the services, as well as changes in the design of the program. Clients accomplished this by developing alliances with political groups, primarily unions. Not only did they attain their goals but they also earned a great deal of respect for their efforts and success.

Incidentally, here is an instance where the eventual contract was written in language that encourages the agency to assist a client group to develop a component of the services. The contracting agency has three years to spin off a fully autonomous client-run community project. A new autonomous nonprofit corporation, which includes many of the clients who protested the award of the contract to the other agency, is being developed to operate part of the program that evolved out of their intervention. Should it turn out that the client group is not able to operate that component of the contracted services at the end of three years, another parent agency will be awarded the contract to complete the development of the new corporation.

If clients are to be given the opportunity to develop their opinions and take control of aspects of the mental health system, mental health planners, program administrators, and clinicians must be open to playing new roles in a more collaborative effort. And clients must attend to the difficulties that had previously led them along self-defeating or isolating paths so that they can play their part in the current collaboration.

Of course, part of the providers' role will be to monitor the collaboration, much as they monitor their own clinical role via peer review. There is an extremely high potential for exploitation of clients and their newfound power. Sometimes charismatic, self-serving individuals will find a way to exploit the vast amount of energy that is unleashed by the client group. With the evolution of truly collaborative programs, the providers and consumers must find some way to prevent this kind of exploitation.

The Story of One Client-Driven Program

In one county where the department of mental health had been contracting with a private, nonprofit agency to provide a transitional housing program (the transition being between an acute residential program serving as an alternative to hospitalization and independent living), the county decided to shift its support to an assisted independent living project in which the clients would play a greater role in servicing the daily needs of their own community members. The new program would require a lower staff-to-client ratio, and therefore the same funds would provide for the housing of more clients.

As part of the project, the county wanted the agency to set up a "respite" within the program's geographic area. It was planned that there would be 75 to 100 clients living in close proximity to each other in the assisted independent living project. The county mental health department asked the director of the agency to set up one apartment with three beds in the midst of the client community to serve as a fully staffed respite for clients who needed a safe place to go. Essentially, this would be a step short of clients going to the county's crisis clinic, the respite apartment thus serving to prevent a certain number of more serious crises.

The administrator of the agency was reluctant to develop the respite component. He believed that to have a designated place for those in crisis to stay and presumably have staff there around the clock or on call to care for them would create the dependency on institutions that the overall program was established to combat. The issue became a topic of discussion in the county and among the clients in the program. After dialogue between the mental health department and the agency, it was determined that having clients plan and staff the program themselves would deal directly with the issue of dependency, while avoiding the problem of clients withdrawing from peers and turning to professional experts whenever they felt they were in crisis. Responsibility for the development of the program was then turned over to the client group. The client group established the guidelines for the use of their respite program, the circumstances that would lead to a client using the facility, how the facility should be supplied, and how many staff should be available. The final issue was staffing. And here was an unanticipated outcome. The clients agreed that they should staff the program, but as unpaid volunteers on a rotating basis. They believed they should care for each other as part of the responsibility of being members of a community. In this instance, clients' input was taken seriously, and they were given the time they required to develop their design for the respite service. This assisted not only in the design but also increased the likelihood that clients who find themselves in crisis will feel safe utilizing the respite and can avoid a dependency-creating system. As long as the group maintains stability, the respite service will be utilized as they designed it.

This development occurred because the agency administrator allowed the clients to control program planning. Clients eventually took control and helped direct the services to meet their needs. The result is that the clients, as a group, gained strength. The administrator's openness to the process and his willingness to give up control in determining an outcome are qualities that mark a good administrator in this age of client-driven programs. If the concept of client-consumer participation in the design and implementation of community mental health services is to be anything more than lip service, then mental health managers and providers must use all their expertise and talent to create an environment that fosters the evolution of client-directed services. And if client groups are given sufficient time and a supportive, safe environment in which to grow and assume control of their programs, then consumers will become a great resource to the mental health system.

References

Bloom, B., and Asher, S. "Patients' Rights and Patient Advocacy: A Historical and Conceptual Appreciation." In B. Bloom and S. Asher (eds.), *Psychiatric Patient Rights and Patient Advocacy*. New York: Human Sciences Press, 1982.

Brown, P. "The Mental Patients' Rights Movement and Mental Health Institutional Change." *International Journal of Health Services*, 1981, *11*, 523–540.

Kupers, T. A. "Advocacy as a Therapeutic Intervention." In T. A. Kupers, *Public Therapy: The Practice of Psychotherapy in the Public Mental Health Clinic*. New York: Free Press, 1981.

Ernest L. Silva is currently an independent consultant to mental health service providers in Northern California.

Those who provide individual and family psychotherapy to inner-city AIDS clients and their families face major treatment challenges.

Therapy with Inner-City AIDS Clients

Lige Dailey, Jr.

In 1987, the Bay Area Black Consortium for Quality Health Care established the AIDS Minority Health Initiative Project (AMHI) to assess the needs and provide case management services to people of color with AIDS-Related Condition (ARC) and AIDS (Hazard, 1989). As part of AMHI's interdisciplinary case management team, which includes a social worker and a public health nurse, I have provided psychotherapy to AIDS clients and their families for the past two years. Although interdisciplinary case management is not a new or unusual approach, psychological intervention as a regular component of case management assessment and ongoing treatment is a relatively new element in the treatment of people with AIDS.

Most of my experience has been in the inner city, working with people whose illnesses are drug related or sexually transmitted. The population served is primarily African American and Mexican American, approximately 50 percent gay and bisexual men, 30 percent heterosexual men, 18 percent heterosexual women, and 2 percent lesbian and bisexual women.

In my entire ten-year career as a psychotherapist, I have yet to encounter clients with as wide a range of treatment needs as my inner-city minority AIDS clients. This population is generally homeless, unemployable, rejected by their families, and shunned by social service agencies. Work with these clients is often stressful and frustrating. It involves negotiating with an endless host of bureaucratic social service providers.

It requires constantly educating providers about the reality and the threat of the AIDS epidemic; for instance, many do not understand the AIDS infection cycle and the early debilitating effects that this deadly virus can have on the AIDS victim's mental and physical functioning. Some do not realize that inner-city drug users, children, and heterosexual men and women are quickly replacing male homosexuals as the population most at risk and that providers must adapt their procedures to fit these changing demographics. Working with minority AIDS clients is a protracted struggle. It has catapulted me into police stations, social service offices, and the homes and hospital rooms of my clients. I have attended courtroom hearings, consciousness-raising rallies, fund raisers, birthday celebrations, and too many funerals.

The AIDS infection carries with it an enormous stigma in inner-city minority communities. There is not a great amount of sympathy for drug users with AIDS from people who have been victimized by drug-related crimes. Nor is there any significant support for gay men whose life-styles have embarrassed their families. Many of these families are frightened, angry, and confused about how to react to the AIDS epidemic. The AIDS virus has spontaneously activated religious biases, issues of personal safety, and family responsibility and pride. It has also created an immediate challenge to inner-city mental health practitioners. I share the following experiences with the hope that they may in some constructive way assist other professionals involved in this struggle.

This chapter will emphasize the inherent treatment challenges and common clinical issues connected with providing psychological services to inner-city minority AIDS clients and their families. By family I mean not only the biological family of origin but also the extended family of choice. This may include friends, lovers, and associates. Throughout this chapter, vignettes will be used to examine the following topics: the psychodynamics of the AIDS infection cycle, the psychosocial obstacles associated with treatment, the effectiveness of psychotherapy, the family treatment approach, and pathological mourning. In the interest of confidentiality, all detailed personal descriptions have been creatively altered to preserve the anonymity of the clients.

The Psychodynamics of the AIDS Infection Cycle

As a result of my ethnographic research and clinical observations, I have come to use certain conceptual treatment approaches that have helped structure my work with AIDS clients and their families. I have identified what appears to be an interrelationship between the AIDS infection cycle and the psychodynamic challenges of Kübler-Ross's (1969) stages of dying. The corresponding phases are as follows:

AIDS Infection Cycle	*Kübler-Ross's Stages*
1. Diagnosed HIV positive: asymptomatic	Denial/"No, not me." (shock/tries to forget)
2. AIDS-related conditions: opportunistic diseases	Rage and anger/"Why me?" (strong emotion)
3. Chronic AIDS: hospitalizations	Bargaining/"Yes me, but . . ." (bargain for extra time)
4. Terminal illness: death watch	Depression and acceptance/ "Yes me." (preparatory grief)
5. The family's bereavement: funerals as a cathartic rite of passage	The family's grief/pathological mourning or acceptance?

The relationships shown in this list are not hard and fast, and there may be exceptions, but in general, knowledge of these phases of disease and dying helps in planning treatment.

My first story is about a twenty-nine-year-old black homosexual man who reported that he knew, in hindsight, that he had AIDS because of the fact that several of his sexual partners had ARC. He was too fearful to be tested. To himself, he rationalized that if he did not think or talk about it, he would not contract the disease. When he finally got up the nerve to be tested, he went to a white testing site so he would not risk running into someone he knew. Clearly, he was in denial. He only came in for psychological evaluation after he had developed symptoms of ARC. Only then did he begin a course of psychotherapy, go through a stage of asking "Why me?", get in touch with the rage he felt about being sick, and eventually, after a course of individual and family therapy, work through his depression and enter the acceptance phase. The last was reflected in his regular attendance at appointments with his medical doctor and with his therapist and in his remorse about having waited so long to be tested and possibly having infected others. Ideally, the aim of psychological treatment is to help the client work through his or her depression and enter the stage of acceptance; at the same time, the psychotherapist must strive not to allow hope to die before the client does. In this case, the terminal illness of the AIDS infection cycle coincided with the acceptance stage in Kübler-Ross's schema.

Psychosocial Obstacles Associated with Treatment

Psychotherapy with black clients during the asymptomatic HIV-positive stage is rare. The majority of the clients I've treated began therapy during the onset of ARC or in the chronic AIDS stage. Based on my experience, I would say that black clients, with or without AIDS, have a noted resistance to early medical or therapeutic interventions. This resistance can probably be correlated to their socioeconomic status and past negative experiences, as well as to ethnic differences.

Many of my clients have reported trying a variety of home remedies and faith healings before surrendering themselves for hospital treatment. Baker, Wright, Mergerson, and Gonick (1953) viewed the decision to seek medical help as a complex conflict involving five separate factors. These included the severity of the symptom, the anticipation of a return to health through treatment, the person's view of himself or herself as a healthy individual not needing medical care, the person's recognition that a trip to the physician may disclose illnesses, and such negative aspects of diagnosis and treatment as cost.

In addition to these factors "within" the individual, help seeking is influenced by the individual's past negative experiences. Many of my clients complain about the ridiculous amounts of time one has to spend in the county hospital waiting to be seen by a physician. They claim that emergency services are a "joke." One particular client felt himself ill and went to the hospital emergency services for treatment. After waiting for almost four hours, he became fatigued and returned home to rest. The next day he called our office and requested a ride to the hospital. We took him to the hospital, and he was admitted. He died the following day. My clients inform me that incidents such as these have caused them to distrust county hospitals and doctors. They were especially distrustful of interns and felt that these young doctors were incompetent and only "practiced on the black and poor" to improve their skills for the rich.

Even when the patient is seen by an experienced physician, there can be significant distrust. I have witnessed interactions between doctors and clients that in my assessment contribute to this distrust and disrespect. Cartwright (1964) lists the following possible reasons for the lack of trust felt by many black patients: Doctors do not expect members of the working class to ask questions and consequently do not encourage questions; skilled and unskilled workers do not know the meaning of technical terms used by doctors; these patients hold physicians in awe; the social distance between the upper-class physician and the working-class patient is too great; and—the most hotly denied—doctors may exhibit a subtle or not-so-subtle racism.

On the other hand, there are many physicians who are dedicated to providing high-quality care to minorities and AIDS sufferers and who are sensitive to the issues listed by Cartwright. Even in these cases, however, patients may feel distrust and may, as a result, be noncompliant with treatment. This may be because the dying patient's expression of anger, the most natural of responses to his or her own death, effectively closes off communication with those professionals offering care (Quint, 1967; Kübler-Ross, 1969).

In any case, the nature and quality of my clients' relationships with their doctors has had a burdensome effect on the psychological work I do with them. Because clients routinely see medical doctors before starting psychotherapy, they often displace their distrust of doctors and hospitals onto me.

The Effectiveness of Psychotherapy

I have found psychotherapy, "the talking cure," to be effective in working with our justifiably suspicious AIDS clients. I have discovered that because these clients have encountered an all-too-common combination of racism, homophobia, and class bias, they are starved for regular, honest, nonjudgmental dialogue and feedback. In therapy sessions, which might have to occur over the phone, in the client's home, on a medical ward, or while walking down the street with the client, the client talks about his or her problems, experiences, attitudes, and feelings. The psychotherapist, in turn, inquires, comments, clarifies, and perhaps advises. From this regular exchange, a bond of mutual trust can be established. The client is then able to understand and manage his or her destructive impulses, thoughts, and actions better. Kübler-Ross (1969), Neugarten (1977), and Levine (1984) believe approaching death can be an opportunity for growth through psychotherapy. According to Neugarten, "awareness of approaching death should perhaps not be viewed as a signal for dissolution of the personality structure, but instead as an impetus for a new and final restructuring" (p. 386).

The Family Treatment Approach

Often individual therapy is not enough. AIDS clients feel a need to make peace with their families. Whether their estrangement resulted from their sexual preference or from intravenous drug use, or whether their leave-taking was problematic for some other reason, they need to interact with their family in a new way before they die.

Research on the families of AIDS victims has been relatively sparse, particularly regarding drug-using populations. A conservative estimate might be that for every person who is infected with the virus, as with any terminal disease, at least five family members are directly and irrevocably affected. Given the projected statistics for AIDS infection over the next several years, a significant number of family members will require a variety of community-based psychosocial services in the nineties.

I have found systemic family therapy (Ackerman, 1970) to be a useful modality for dealing with the intrapsychic, interpersonal, and psychosocial dimensions of AIDS. Ackerman noticed that successes in individual psychoanalysis were often undermined when the client returned to the family environment. He began treating the whole family, believing that all aspects of a client's existence were of equal importance. With AIDS clients, there are a number of issues that regularly arise in terms of the family. These include leftover issues about the way the adult child originally separated from the family, unresolved sibling rivalry, child abuse, domestic violence, and leftover resentment about drug use or homosexual life-style. The next vignette illustrates some of these themes.

The AIDS death watch is gradually becoming an identifiable family syndrome. The mother of a forty-two-year-old black AIDS victim sobbed almost uncontrollably over the telephone. Finally, she was able to say, "I know this sounds horrible, but what's taking my daughter so long to die? She's causing our family terrible problems. I can't sleep, I can't eat, and I have constant headaches. She's not satisfied with my home care and has begun to curse me. It's becoming difficult not to hate her . . . but she's sick and still my child. Her friends are bringing her dope to use in my home, and her sisters and brothers aren't helping me as they promised. I feel guilty for complaining, but I feel trapped! I never felt so helpless before. I'm becoming more angry and depressed each day. I'm beginning to feel more of a victim of AIDS than my daughter."

An alarming number of families who provide home care to intravenous drug users and homosexuals dying of AIDS are calling on community mental health professionals to mediate disputes and stresses caused by the presence of the person with AIDS. In many cases, it is the mother who finds herself in an impossible dilemma. She is horrified by the fact that she feels frustration and dissatisfaction that her terminally ill son or daughter has not expired in a timely manner. Strong anger and guilt usually immobilize the family and transform them into passive-aggressive martyrs. Predictably, the person with AIDS capitalizes on this situation and seeks revenge from the family for having earlier rejected him or her because of a homosexual or drug-abusing life-style.

In this case, after the physician informed the family that this woman was terminally ill and had less than two months to live, the family felt it their duty to invite her to return home to die. In fact, she lived almost a year. It was as if the family, in the face of her impending death, had forgotten who this woman really was—for instance, that she was selfish, manipulative, uncooperative, and capable of stealing from them to support her habit. Then, when the two months had passed and she was not only still alive and a burden but also bringing her drug-using friends home, the family was forced to confront the kinds of conflicts that had originally led to their kicking her out of the house.

It was only after she had been home for five months that the family sought help from our interdisciplinary treatment team. We conducted a home visit to evaluate the problem. After members of the team had spoken with each family member individually, it became apparent that the family had overcommitted itself and would be unable to care for its sick member. The family, as so often happens, was idealizing its dying relative, a form of pathological mourning. In addition, the patient was experiencing some dementia, and the woman's memory loss created further problems. In short, this family did not have the resources to care for this woman at home, but the family members' guilt made it impossible to turn her away. Then, when she acted badly, they were enraged but felt guilty about that reaction.

I conducted a series of family therapy sessions with the immediate family. The sick woman spoke about her need for more medical care, her physical pain, and her frustration with the family's inability to provide for her. Other family members spoke of their frustration in trying to meet her constant demands and the pain they felt watching her die. She shared that accepting her eventual death was difficult and made her angry with the world. I reframed the problem, telling them that at this stage of the illness, she really required more medical support than the family could supply and that she should consider going to a hospice. Once inside the hospice, she could have twenty-four-hour medical care, and the family could visit on a regular basis. In fact, the family would be able to take care of many needs that the staff could not satisfy, such as responding to special food requests and taking her to church. They all agreed to the plan. During the two weeks it took to locate a hospice that was willing to accept someone who acted out in the way that this woman did, we visited the family several times at home. The woman with AIDS was then moved to a hospice. Through continuing psychotherapy and family support, she was able to advance to the acceptance stage and died peacefully three months later.

In this case, our job was first to help the family recognize the reality of its limitations and to support its dying relative in the most constructive way possible, without allowing her illness to destroy them all. Then, after the move and the woman's eventual death, the treatment involved working through grief and guilt about abandoning a sick family member.

There are advantages to working with an interdisciplinary team. It is helpful to collaborate during the initial assessment and adoption of a therapeutic strategy. It helps to have several providers get to know the family. Sometimes particular family members are able to confide in one member of the team but not in another. Sometimes two therapists are needed as cotherapists with the family, or the team might decide that one member should conduct individual therapy and another family therapy. Sometimes team members, perhaps ones who are not directly involved in the psychotherapy, can help the therapists sort out countertransference dilemmas and stalemates in treatment. And I personally find it invaluable to have the support of team members in this difficult work.

Pathological Mourning

Mourning is an active process. Coping with loss requires work, whether it is the loss of a loved one or the realization that one is going to die. Pathological mourning occurs when the active process is blocked. Instead of the work of mourning, there are symptoms (Lindemann, 1944): social isolation, hypochondriasis, paranoia, agitated depression, psychotic decompensation, or other symptoms. The symptoms might be mild or severe.

A thirty-five-year-old Latino homosexual man from out of state came to my office seemingly obsessed about "being unemployed and broke." In spite of the fact that he was afraid of being "penniless," I saw him flag a cab on several occasions, and he was able to withdraw a certain amount of money from a bank savings account when he needed to. During the first few months of individual psychotherapy, while he complained repeatedly about his economic status, he was able to find one job after another but was unable to keep any of the jobs. In explaining his inability to keep these jobs, he would list complaints about his employers: They don't pay enough, they're not professional, they're not businesslike, and so on. There seemed to be some paranoid distortions in his reporting of events.

This man was suffering from ARC, which he told me at the beginning of treatment. In the first few months of therapy, however, he did not want to talk about that or about his feelings about being sick. Slowly, he began to talk in glowing terms about an ex-lover. He brought in a picture of the man and spoke of their love relationship. As he became a little more trusting, he shared that he was also angry at the man, not only because he (the ex-lover) had died of AIDS but also because he had not mentioned my client in his will. As the idealization of the ex-lover diminished, he told me that half of the couple's furniture had belonged to him, but because his lover had owned the house, the dead man's family (who had disapproved of the homosexual relationship) had been able to lock up the house and deny him access to his rightful belongings. In addition, he believed he had contracted the AIDS virus from his ex-lover, who had also betrayed him by being sexually unfaithful.

As the idealization disappeared and there was more trust within the therapeutic relationship, he began to confide that two new lovers reminded him of his ex-lover—in fact, he actually believed they were his ex-lover reincarnated. One of these new lovers was confined to a wheelchair, and this client believed that physical disability represented a punishment for the ex-lover's betrayal. In other words, this man was experiencing delusions. He began to say more about his feelings for his ex-lover. When asked if he might be feeling some anger, he became enraged about the betrayal. Then, when I suggested that he might have mixed feelings and also be really missing him, he broke down and cried for the first time since his ex-lover's death. The delusions receded, and he shared the insight that he did not really want to let his ex-lover go. He continued to cry and grieve, and over the ensuing months, he reported less distrust and very little delusional material. He eventually was able to find a job, and his concerns about money decreased in magnitude. He was now free to process the psychodynamics of his own impending deterioration and eventual death from AIDS. Thus, the symptoms of pathological mourning—delusions, idealization, and isolation—cleared up as the man was able to actively grieve.

Conclusion

I have attempted to describe how, when working with clients with ARC or AIDS, I have found it useful to consider the relationship between the infection cycle and Kübler-Ross's stages of death and dying. This work is best achieved through the knowledge and application of psychodynamic principles and techniques. The family treatment approach should also be considered as the appropriate way to include the significant people in a client's life, whether these people are part of a family of biological origin or one of choice. It is vital to the AIDS client that these significant others find a place in our overall treatment strategies.

I know from experience that interdisciplinary team case management works. Its effectiveness, however, depends heavily on the team members' ability to develop interpersonal treatment alliances with clients. When such alliances are established, collaboration can begin and a support system is in place to help clients and their families through the time of the client's death and to help families in the aftermath.

Finally, the obstacles that compromise treatment—such as racism, homophobia, class bias, and ignorance—must be constantly challenged. AIDS is caused by a relatively newly evolved virus that presents tough challenges to our medical competence. The bigger problem may be that at this point it appears that the virus is more willing to change its form than we are to change the social realities that make it so dangerous.

References

Ackerman, N. W. "Family Psychotherapy and Psychoanalysis: Implications of Difference." In N. W. Ackerman (ed.), *Family Process*. New York: Basic Books, 1970.

Baker, R. G., Wright, B. A., Mergerson, L., and Gonick, M. R. *Adjustment to*

Physical Handicap and Illness: A Survey of the Social Psychology of Physique and Disability. (2nd ed.) New York: Social Science Research Council, 1953.

Cartwright, A. *Human Relations and Hospital Care.* London: Routledge & Kegan Paul, 1964.

Hazard, M. *AIDS Minority Health Initiative Case Management Policies and Procedures.* Oakland, Calif.: Bay Area Black Consortium for Quality Health Care, 1989.

Kübler-Ross, E. *On Death and Dying.* New York: Macmillan, 1969.

Levine, S. *Meetings at the Edge: Dialogues with the Grieving and Dying, the Healing and the Healed.* New York: Doubleday, 1984.

Lindemann, E. "Symptomatology and Management of Acute Grief." *American Journal of Psychiatry,* 1944, *101,* 141–148.

Neugarten, L. "Personality and Aging." In J. E. Birren and K. W. Schaie (eds.), *Handbook of the Psychology of Aging.* New York: Van Nostrand Reinhold, 1977.

Quint, J. G. *The Nurse and the Dying Patient.* New York: Macmillan, 1967.

Lige Dailey, Jr., is currently the counseling coordinator of the AIDS Minority Health Initiative Project and the counseling coordinator of Parental Stress Services in Oakland, California.

A combination of individual and family therapies is utilized
by staff and trainees to handle difficult cases in the child and
adolescent outpatient clinic of an inner-city hospital.

A Multimodality Approach to the Treatment of Children and Families

Herbert A. Schreier

The Family Guidance Clinic, as the child psychiatry unit at Children's Hospital of Oakland is called, receives an average of one new request per day for consultation from the medical or surgical inpatient units of the hospital, and five times that number of outpatient requests. The cases may involve crises stemming from the recent drug wars in Oakland, or they may involve complicated symptomatology, since the hospital has become a referral center for the entire area. It does not take any intricate calculations to figure out that we are inundated with cases requiring psychotherapy, both individual and family. In this chapter, I will describe our multimodality approach to therapy with an inner-city population and then discuss the pragmatics of operating a clinic in the inner city.

The Use of Multiple Modalities

Unlike some groups who have lined up behind one form of therapy or another, we choose our modalities based on how much the family will tolerate, the resources of the clinic, and the skill of the therapist. We conduct trainings for clinicians in a variety of modalities, in some cases using one or another for most of the therapeutic encounter. We also keep an eye on the family's tendency to flee when a modicum of stability has been introduced. We have found that structural family therapy with the emphasis it places on "joining" with the family helps form early bonds that can be called on in the "flight into health" stage of treatment (Minuchin, 1974). We are also not above calling on the child's pediatrician, school, or social agencies for help in keeping the families in therapy.

The advantage of the multimodality approach, aside from what we consider its direct usefulness, is that it stimulates a reasonably high level of excitement, an interchange of ideas, and a lively debate in what might otherwise become, given the "heaviness" of the cases, a fairly maudlin atmosphere. Every case is presented in the staff's weekly rounds session, with ideas flowing fairly freely. These sessions are augmented by ones where staff members present their work on videotape to other staff and to students. It is rewarding to watch our "impossible" cases improve.

We do not insist that every therapist in the clinic be able to handle all modalities. Colleagues might be called in for their particular strengths or interests, and sometimes supervisory changes are made in the middle of therapy.

Using our multimodality approach, even trainees with a background in psychoanalytic psychotherapy may eventually become comfortable making a paradoxical prescription for a hospital patient whom we have been given a mere two days to "cure." This "firing-line" atmosphere tends to lead us toward a judicious and respectful use of psychotropic medications. For instance, an anxious boy acts out at school because he fears for the safety of a hypertensive, overweight single mother who lives in a drive-by shoot-up neighborhood and who is depressed. The school gives us two weeks to improve his behavior, or they will insist that he be put on home tutoring. We prescribe Imipramine, which helps a great deal, and meanwhile we are able to work at a more leisurely pace with the family.

In order to illustrate our general approach, I will briefly describe two representative cases and discuss aspects of the treatments.

Calvin and His Family. Calvin Green, a fifteen-and-a-half-year-old African American boy, was referred to the Family Guidance Clinic at Children's Hospital during an inpatient admission for asthma because a psychologically minded resident physician took a history of school failure, truancy, and fighting, as well as of difficulties at home that were felt to be related to the impending death of his stepfather. His half-brother (age six), his half-sister (age eight), and the mother (age thirty-two) came in for family sessions. Initially the work focused on Calvin's conflicts with his stepfather, this seventy-year-old man's debilitating illness, and his eventual demise three weeks after the family first came to the clinic. Because the mother was keeping the kids at home and was overtly hostile to the idea of therapy and to the therapist (a white male) and because the sessions were often quite chaotic with Calvin repeatedly threatening suicide, the staff decided to use a structural family approach (Minuchin, 1974). One of the staff psychologists, a black woman, was added to these weekly sessions. Some progress was made through this approach in getting the mother to take responsibility for sending her children to school.

In the third month of therapy, the mother began to miss sessions, and the school again reported numerous absences even though the children were not in other kinds of trouble. When the student therapist, at the urging of the supervisor, pursued the mother by phone, she returned with the children. In a tearful segment of a session, while alone with the therapist, the mother revealed that she had given birth to Calvin just prior to serving a two-year jail sentence. On her release, she had picked Calvin up from her sister and brother-in-law, and she had been devastated by his rejection of her.

At this point, the staff felt that the tenor of the family work needed to shift, and they decided to use a combination of structural work and what has come to be known as object-relations family therapy (Scharff and Scharff, 1987). The focus became the mother's internal representation of the patient and his siblings. She was seen separately during parts of several of the family sessions. The following history reemerged, a history that had been gathered in the earlier sessions but that had been presented at that time with minimal affect: The mother had been sexually abused by her father and subsequently rejected by her mother when she revealed this; she had turned then to prostitution and drugs, which had led to her jail sentence. This time her tears and affect seemed to fit the story she was telling.

When the case was presented to me in the course of a videotaped family therapy seminar, it became clear that an intense erotic transference was developing with the male student therapist. This was related to the mother's resistance, which took the form of making verbal attacks, keeping secrets from the therapist, and attempting to flee therapy again. The transference also seemed to be causing some anxiety in the therapist. Because the current family supervisor felt uncomfortable with the more dynamic turn this course of family therapy was taking, we decided that I would take over supervision of the case, and we would review videotapes of each weekly session. As the work intensified, the mother again tried to flee and missed sessions. We decided that the therapist should contact the school and Calvin's doctors, thereby putting pressure on Mom to return with the kids for family therapy.

Shapiro and Carr (1987) present a model for using the same therapist as a family therapist as well as an individual dynamic therapist, a model they have applied successfully in an inpatient setting at McClain's Hospital in Boston. We were essentially adapting that model in an outpatient setting. In individual sessions, the mother's transference reactions were explored. The therapist brought insights, such as the ability to predict how Mom would react toward her children, from the individual sessions into the family sessions without revealing the confidences of the individual sessions. As this lessened the chances of the mother's acting out, more positive feelings were able to emerge from the children, who were now returning to school in a fairly steady way. In the mother's intense individual brief therapy with "others in the room" (Gustafson, 1986), she was able to develop considerable insight into the therapeutic relationship. She was proud of this "newfound ability" to understand rather than to act out, and she began to see therapy as a collaborative effort. Trust in another, even one (the therapist) who was going to leave in just two short months, was proving worth her effort. The therapist's anxieties diminished accordingly.

Lamar and His Mother. Lamar Stanton's mother called because she felt that her sixteen-year-old son was "seriously suicidal." Lamar had never known his biological father, who was black. His Caucasian mother, who had been ostracized by her own upper-class North Carolina family, had moved to California with Lamar soon after leaving her husband, who had been physically and verbally abusive to both of them. The young man had become suicidal and was hospitalized for two weeks. Then his ambivalent mother signed him out against medical advice. But he returned to the clinic for outpatient family therapy. The student intern was at first intimidated by this young man's leaving the sessions early, smashing furniture and walls, and in general intimidating both her and his mother. With guidance from her supervisor, the therapist was able to set the tenets of her former analytic training aside and insist that the patient needed to stay in therapy and needed to stay in the room. (I am reminded of Harry Aponte's dictum: "If I don't get simple I cry" [Aponte, 1986]). After some "structure" was brought to the family, the therapist was able to explore with them their family dynamics, while providing support for the mother and more intensive individual dynamic work for the son in individual sessions with each of them. In the space of ten months, the therapist was able to apply these different modalities and reach a resolution, which allowed for the peaceful separation of this dyad in what could be considered a reasonably appropriate manner.

Intensive psychotherapy takes time, and in mental health settings, time is money. When working with low-income inner-city children and families, therapists cannot always collect fees for their services. Consequently some creative financing is indicated. A discussion of our therapeutic approach would not be complete without some mention of the way our program runs.

The Operation of the Clinic

The Family Guidance Clinic was started in the late fifties as the private nonprofit hospital began to change from a small community hospital to one with a large subspecialty care and training responsibility. The part-time director of the Child Psychiatry Service prior to my arrival had been working with five part-time psychologists and social workers and one student. While the clinic staff saw children from the inner city surrounding the hospital, they also saw inpatients for consultation and were responsible for teaching the interns and residents about behavioral difficulties. In the twenty-five years since that time, the hospital has nearly doubled in bed capacity, and its tertiary-care role (i.e., specialty hospital) now includes fifty-two beds for an intensive care nursery, sixteen beds for oncology, fifteen for rehabilitative medicine, and twenty-five for intensive care. The hospital is one of only fourteen national pediatric trauma centers. There are now 110 physicians on staff, many of them subspecialists in pediatrics, and seventy interns and residents.

Parallel to the general trend in mental health care, the Family Guidance Clinic staff has increased by only one full-time equivalent over the last eleven years. We compensate for the staff shortage and handle the dramatically increasing need for psychological services by expanding our student group to between fifteen and seventeen child psychology students, child psychiatry fellows, social workers, and mental health workers.

Though we have increased "productivity" enormously, the clinic continues to lose a substantial sum of money for the hospital. Medi-Cal (California's Medicaid), the major third-party payer for the clinic, will pay well below cost for a visit and then only for every-other-week sessions, clearly not adequate for the cases described here. Numerous studies demonstrating that adequate psychological services for chronically ill children and their families can dramatically reduce hospital stays have fallen on the same deaf ears that ignore studies showing that aggressive outreach prenatal care costing pennies can prevent long stays in our neonatal ICU, where costs reach $1,800 to $2,000 a day.

The hospital tolerates the Family Guidance Clinic's deficit partly because of a sense of community obligation and partly as a service to its physician community. Children's Hospital trains most of the area's pediatricians who work both in middle-class areas and inner-city ghettos surrounding the hospital. These physicians have come to see the department as a resource for their most difficult patients. Further, we have convinced the administration that our large size is necessary if we are to provide quick responses to inpatient consultations, to teach, and to prevent staff burnout. We have been helped in this cause by two administrators whose sensitivity to the importance of intensive psychological services is high indeed.

It is within this context that our clinical approach has evolved over my eleven years at Children's Hospital. The context is similar in some ways to community mental health centers but different in some important regards. Unlike community mental health centers, we can select whom we choose to see, as the requests for service far exceed our capacity. We also see a range of children from the various socioeconomic strata. Though some 80 percent of our clients are poor, they are highly motivated to participate in the clinic's programs. Our use of students means that staff have time to teach without enormous pressure to see more and more cases. Research opportunities are also generated by our psychology graduate students and often involve staff members. Finally, working in a large medical center provides a range of interesting problems in diagnosis, treatment, liaison work, and research that are not always found in clinics located in the community.

Conclusion

This work can be rewarding as well as exciting. No one can do this work alone. Our work is varied and involves teaching therapy as well as our own continued learning. Our clients seem to understand that we are serious about providing psychotherapy. The clinic's rate of failed appointments is somewhere around 10 percent. In times of diminished resources for public mental health services, parts of our model might find ready acceptance in community mental health clinics.

The nation's medical system is under attack for being costly and comparatively ineffective. When "cost-saving" programs are instituted, the poor and mentally ill suffer disproportionately. Psychiatry, never luxuriantly supported, will find the resources allotted it even further diminished. The model I have described is pragmatic in its approach, as we have adjusted to years of underfunding by setting short-, medium-, and long-term therapeutic goals. Knowing that we couldn't possibly take care of all the problems presented to us has actually helped us to set these goals. It is not obvious to us that longer treatment is as frequently indicated for therapeutic reasons as the mode in the private sector would suggest. With others who have written about brief therapy, we feel that there is often a benefit to having a focused, time-limited approach (Malan, 1976, and Gustafson, 1986).

References

Aponte, H. J. "If I Don't Get Simple I Cry." *Family Process*, 1986, *25*, 531–548.
Gustafson, J. P. *The Complex Secret of Brief Psychotherapy*. New York: Norton, 1986.
Malan, D. *The Frontier of Brief Psychotherapy*. London: Plenum, 1976.
Minuchin, S. *Families and Family Therapy*. Cambridge, Mass.: Harvard University Press, 1974.
Scharff, D. E., and Scharff, J. S. *Object-Relations Family Therapy*. Northvale, N.J.: Aronson, 1987.
Shapiro, E. R., and Carr, A. W. "Disguised Countertransference in Institutions." *Psychiatry*, 1987, *50*, 72–82.

Herbert A. Schreier is chief of family guidance services at Children's Hospital in Oakland, California.

As public psychiatry programs for the elderly begin to emerge, we must refine our therapeutic theories and techniques in order to serve this population better.

Psychotherapy with the Elderly in Public Mental Health Settings

Carl I. Cohen

In the past, older persons have been poorly served by public psychiatry. Persons aged sixty-five and over receive only 4 percent of services rendered by community mental health centers (U.S. General Accounting Office, 1982), despite comprising 12 percent of the population and having levels of psychopathology comparable to those of younger persons (Myers and others, 1984). During the era of rapid deinstitutionalization, many aged individuals were shunted to nursing homes, most of which lacked adequate mental health services (Talbott, 1987). However, as the number of older persons continues to grow dramatically, we have seen an increased advocacy on the part of older psychiatric patients and their families, a heightened professional sensitivity toward aging, proliferation of geriatric psychiatrists and other trained professionals, some improvements in Medicare reimbursement for psychiatric services, a modification in nursing home regulations to ensure adequate psychiatric care, and the development of model mental health programs for at-risk elderly. The confluence of these events should help spawn an expansion of services for the elderly in the decades to come. Thus, this is a propitious time in which to consider what forms therapy might take for the elderly served in public mental health settings.

Much of psychodynamic theory and technique was developed with relatively young, predominantly white middle-class Europeans and Americans who were generally well educated. It is not clear how relevant these theories and practices are to therapy with the elderly in public settings. When Freud ([1904]1957) proclaimed that psychoanalysis is not very effective for analysands over fifty, he was suggesting that past a certain age people tend to be set in their ways and not very willing to change. Modern therapists have proved Freud wrong in regard to the flexibility of elders. But there are other problems with using the traditional model of psychotherapy in the public sector. Halleck (1971) reflects that those therapists who work solely with the individual patient are prone to minimize or neglect the familial and social spheres. This kind of neglect makes psychotherapy ineffectual with elders if only because familial and social concerns become much more important with age, and this is especially true for those in the lower socioeconomic strata—namely, those served by public mental health programs. If psychotherapy is to be effective, public therapists must pay close attention to the social realities that determine the circumstances and the quality of life of elders.

In this chapter, I will discuss several key issues—the loss of a previous social role, the concomitants of class status and race, the fall into dependency, and a reliance on medications—that underlie some of the symptomatology (such as depression) in the elderly and that must be taken into consideration (along with all the psychodynamic issues that are at issue with any age group) by the therapist if psychotherapy is to be effective. Then I will move on to consider the nontraditional therapeutic modalities of network analysis and social action.

Aging and Loss of Role

In many ways, old age is a socially created category (Estes, Swan, and Gerard, 1984). While it is true that physical and mental decline accelerate in old age, the rates vary by individual (Rowe and Kahn, 1987) and in no way correspond to age sixty-five, which is the benchmark of aging in our society. At age sixty-five, most people are forced into a new social status, that of dependency. Although new laws prohibit age discrimination and mandatory retirement, the availability of Social Security, various pensions, and retirement incentives conspire to extrude the older worker. An entire field—gerontology—has mushroomed around assessing service needs and providing services to the elderly. This social dependency affects the elderly in various ways. Because they are nonproductive, they are thought to be superfluous; they are "blamed" for creating an economic drain on younger workers; negative stereotypes appear in the media; and older individuals incorporate these societal views into their self-images.

I will briefly present two cases where the loss of role plays an important part in the etiology of symptoms. Mr. H. is a black, sixty-six-year-old retired factory worker. He was happy to leave his job on an assembly line, although he and his wife must now live on his very modest Social Security check and pension. Furthermore, he has been under severe strain because he must help care for his ninety-one-year-old mother, and his two teenage granddaughters have been living in his apartment because their mother (his daughter) has a drug problem. When he worked, he used to "let off steam" with some of the other men after work—having a few beers, going to ball games, or shooting some pool. Since he stopped work, he hardly ever sees them. He doesn't have a car, nor does he have the time or desire to go see any of them. Mr. H. developed a series of physical complaints, including headaches, chest pain, and intestinal cramps. Physical examination failed to reveal any pathology. Although Mr. H. minimized his depression, he was referred to a psychiatrist. Because of the 50 percent copayment charge and the limited number of visits covered by Medicare, the psychiatrist could only offer Mr. H. medication and supportive therapy on a monthly basis. After several months in treatment, Mr. H. showed some improvement, but many symptoms, as well as the underlying depression, remained.

Ms. M. is a seventy-year-old lawyer who recently retired after a successful career in a prestigious law firm. Ms. M. regularly visits museums, goes to the theater, and has dinner with her friends. She is able to do this in spite of the fact that her husband is suffering from Alzheimer's disease. Her relative wealth and large apartment enable her to maintain a full-time home-care worker for her husband. Ms. M. initially felt depressed and had difficulty dealing with guilt feelings about leaving her husband with someone. She believed this difficulty stemmed from a long-term problem that she had with "duty" and "guilt." She went to a prominent psychotherapist twice a week for six months to help her deal more effectively with these feelings.

In both cases, the individuals experienced a change or loss of role and depressive symptoms, and there was psychotherapeutic intervention. This is not an unusual constellation around the event of retirement. But retirement does not have the same consequences for everyone, as the contrast between the two cases demonstrates. Over his lifetime, Mr. H. had coped by denying or minimizing his psychic pain. Even when he sensed something was wrong, he had neither the resources for nor the access to professional assistance. Perhaps these facts contributed to the surfacing of his depression in physical symptoms. On the other hand, Ms. M. was quite attuned to her psychological states, several of her friends had previously used her psychotherapist, and she viewed therapy as a healthy way to deal with her long-term guilt feelings. All individuals must learn to cope with a role loss when they retire, but the experience is not the same for everyone. Class matters quite a bit.

Importance of Class

Texts on psychotherapy have invariably treated the elderly as a monolithic group. Although lip service may be paid to social context or to potential diversity among the aged (Butler, 1975), the clinician or writer often

brushes these issues aside and focuses on the "universal" aspects of retirement—that is, the aspects that are shared by elders of all classes. For
example, retirement, cognitive decline, dependency, disability, physical
deterioration and disease, social losses, and death are topics commonly
addressed in the clinical literature (Lazarus and Sadavoy, 1988; Sadavoy
and Leszoz, 1987; Yesavage and Karasu, 1982). In proposing therapeutic
strategies for these problems, the authors rarely differentiate the consequences of retirement for the professional from those for the manual
laborer or the effects of dependency and disability on middle- and upper-
class versus lower-class individuals. Each of these items carries the bag-
gage of social class and cultural context. In working with middle- and
upper-class elderly, therapists show a propensity to minimize the impact
of the social context and to focus on intra- and interpersonal issues. Of
course, for the middle class, the aging process confronts individuals with
a financial marginality they never realized was their plight when they
were fit and working. But work with the indigent elderly served by public
psychiatry literally compels the therapist to confront social forces such as
economics and race because of their more apparent effects on patients'
lives. Therefore, in developing an effective psychotherapy for this population, we must consider the influences of the broader social structure.

The therapist must be aware that even minimal cutbacks in social
services can have significant effects on the quality of life, even the survival, of elders in the lower socioeconomic classes. Inflation, rent in-
creases, and illness can all deplete funds. It is estimated that one-fourth
of the elderly live at or near the poverty level (Minkler, 1984). Moreover,
methods for calculating the poverty level are probably inaccurate for
those over sixty-five, and revised estimates place over one-third of the
elderly as living below the poverty level (Navarro, 1984). Among the
elderly, approximately one-half of black aged and two-fifths of unmarried
older women are living at or near the poverty level (Minkler, 1984). Thus,
if therapy is to be relevant to this population, the therapist must avoid
limiting its scope to intrapsychic and interpersonal issues. There are
economic realities and survival issues that require attention. The therapist gains the patient's trust by demonstrating an understanding of such
things and a willingness to talk about them.

A Note About Race

In my experience, older patients will readily point out differences between
their age and the therapist's, but it is rare for them to comment on racial
or class differences. Therapists must encourage verbalization about these
differences when there are indications that there is some reason to explore
the patient's feelings about them, and therapists must be alert to how
such differences may affect therapy, especially through transference and

countertransference. Butts and Schachter (1968) observed that most blacks enter therapy with fear and suspicion, but racial differences can also serve as a catalyst for therapeutic transference. Terestman, Miller, and Weber (1974) noted that it is important for therapists to strive consciously to go beyond class-stereotype views of their patients, to avoid downgrading treatment expectations, not to confuse class or racial factors with traits that may be part of the disorder (such as paranoid delusions in a black individual versus a realistic sense of danger in a social context where racism prevails), and to be alert to ways in which these factors might be used as resistances.

Often it is difficult to isolate the effects of race. Many aged patients in the public mental health system suffer from the triple jeopardy of being poor, minority, and old. Elderly patients served in public settings have probably experienced patterns of racism, worked in marginal jobs interspersed with periods of unemployment, or suffered discrimination or endured hardships because of their sex. Middle and old age has brought physical disease, an intensification of poverty, and loss of many family members and friends. Such experiences have penetrated and influenced the formation of the unconscious, the defenses, the cognitive style, and the personality.

The clinician must make interpretations on several levels. Fanon (1967) suggests that when a black patient describes a dream in which he has become white, the psychotherapist has two obligations to the patient. First, as an analyst, he or she must help the patient become conscious of the unconscious and abandon attempts at a hallucinatory whitening. But second, once this theme has been brought into consciousness, the therapist must put the patient in a position to choose action (or passivity) with respect to the real source of the conflict—that is, toward social events. The clinician has an analogous obligation with elderly patients, particularly those treated in public settings.

The Dependency Problem

Services for older people have generally been built around encouraging dependency. Transportation services, light-chore services, work and volunteer programs, and other programs that might enhance independence are funded at infinitesimally low levels (Kane, Ouslander, and Abrass, 1984). Often persons must accept higher levels of dependency (through congregate care programs or nursing homes, for example) because there are inadequate services in the community.

The passage of Medicare and Medicaid legislation in 1965 has had a profound effect on how health services are delivered to the elderly. The legislation spawned a dramatic growth in the number of hospital beds and nursing homes (Brown, 1984). Nursing homes, although not well reimbursed under Medicare, received substantial compensation through Medicaid. Funding and reimbursement were relatively high for inpatient services and nursing homes, but there was little or no reimbursement for home services and community treatment. (For example, maximum inpatient reimbursement was $250 per year under the original Medicare legislation, and in 1990 maximum reimbursement will be eliminated, but the 50 percent copayment will remain.) Thus, the legislation has had several consequences for mental health delivery for the elderly. People are forced to choose more restrictive settings for care; people have had to impoverish themselves before they could obtain long-term care; outpatient care was limited to only a few sessions, unless the person was eligible for Medicaid; and unlike other medical specialties, psychiatry had caps placed on outpatient Medicare reimbursement, and copayments were made at 50 percent rather than 80 percent. The first and second consequences serve to foster greater dependency.

A somewhat related concern is whether certain types of behaviors would be best viewed as "state" rather than "trait" phenomena (Ryan, 1971). For example, an indigent, arthritic elderly woman who must constantly badger friends and relatives to assist with transportation, shopping, heavy cleaning, and getting to doctors' appointments might be labeled as having a "dependent personality." However, if this woman had sufficient wealth to purchase maid service, car service, and home food deliveries, she would probably not be considered dependent. On the contrary, she might be characterized as a fiercely independent woman who is trying to survive in the community despite her physical handicaps. Thus, state theory views the first woman's behavior as a response to a particular social environment, while trait theory would maintain that her behavior reflected a long-term, characterological pattern of dependency.

Elders tend to have a lot to say about the issue of dependency, but they are rarely given an opportunity to talk with providers about it. The therapist is in a unique position to explore the patient's conflicts about dependency. Sometimes it helps to discuss ways in which the structure of the health and social service systems encourages dependency. Sometimes it is important to support the patient's attempts to remain as independent as possible. And sometimes the therapist must attempt to help the patient adjust to the dependency that is part of his or her condition or circumstances. In each case, it helps to weave the social reality as well as the psychological issues into the discussion.

Medications and Psychotherapy

Another important factor affecting mental health services to the elderly involves our cultural proclivity to rely on medications, especially when alternative treatments are unavailable. After cardiovascular drugs and analgesics, sedatives and hypnotics are the most common type of drugs taken by the elderly (Salzman, 1984). More than half of the patients in skilled nursing homes and 30 percent of the elderly hospitalized for medical-surgical care receive psychotropic medication (Salzman, 1984). The combination of low reimbursement for outpatient treatment, the influence of the pharmaceutical industry's advertising campaigns on clinicians and consumers, and the general negative image about older people has worked to consign the elderly to limited psychotherapeutic endeavors. Although supportive treatment has never been systematically compared to other models, most authors urge the use of this method, often combined with pharmacotherapy (Sadavoy and Leszcz, 1987). It is plausible that therapists create a rationale to justify this treatment strategy because, within the current economic atmosphere, only affluent elderly could afford more time-consuming treatment.

In any case, in therapy, the aim is to place the patient in the position of making choices about the treatment. A thorough education about the medications available, their effects and side effects, and alternative treatments including psychotherapy and social support services is a must if the patient is to be able to make choices. Not infrequently, when the topic is discussed, the elder patient confides in the therapist that he or she knows that overreliance on medications is just a way to keep him or her quiet, but he or she goes along in order not to be even more of a burden to others. Unless the clinician raises the issue of reliance on medications, a whole series of conflicts about self-esteem, guilt, and dependency is likely to be missed.

Limits of Individual Psychotherapy

"Elders are too set in their ways for psychotherapy to work." That myth too often serves as a rationalization for the limitations of mental health services for the elderly, especially in the public sector. In therapy it is possible to confront psychological defenses that contribute to elders' mental suffering and constrict constructive activity. As suggested in the case of Mr. H., some poor and minority elders use denial or repression to help them cope with lifelong stressors and crises; others use alcohol or tranquilizers to help them forget their troubles. Likewise, many patients use displacement and projection to deal with internalized rage. Thus, an elderly woman who has spent a frustrating and debasing morning at the Medicaid office attempting to get reinstated returns home and unleashes a tirade at her grandson over some minor infraction. In confronting these defenses, the therapist simultaneously comes face to face with the psychological conflicts and the social forces that promoted these defenses.

Therapy in the public sector aims to reawaken in the aging patient the hope of changed circumstances. Freire's (1987) statement about the aim of education is relevant: "As an active educational method helps a person to become consciously aware of his context and his condition as a human being as subject, it will become an instrument of choice" (p. 56). Conventional therapeutic strategies often include cognitive and behavioral methods to overcome a patient's belief in his or her helplessness. Such strategies might include graduated tasks, relaxation techniques, physical exercises, and assertiveness training. Because broader social forces must be addressed, especially when working with elderly poor and minority patients, traditional cognitive behavioral approaches may be too limited. Thus, for example, elderly patients who present with depression or anxiety commonly report difficulties with landlords, with governmental agencies, with crime, and with the inadequacy of public transportation. These difficulties impede their ability to visit family and friends, to do their shopping, and to keep medical appointments. The therapist must help the patient identify these social stressors as part of his or her psychological problem. Then, the clinician and patient can develop tactics for tackling these problems; some of the tactics may relate to individual, family, or group therapy, and for some psychotherapy may not suffice. Rather, there is a need for social interventions, such as forming linkages to advocacy groups.

Network Analysis, Social Intervention, and Advocacy

Social structures have created a situation in which the lower-income population primarily served by public therapy has limited options with respect to type and duration of clinical treatment and other supportive services. This is not to say that various therapeutic techniques (such as pharmacotherapy, cognitive behavioral methods, and dynamic therapy) are not useful. But by focusing solely on the individual as the origin of and solution to her or his problems, we neglect broader causes and solutions. Indeed, public psychiatry must go beyond the office and the singular client into the community and the client's social world. Public psychiatry has the opportunity (and the necessity) to develop new perspectives and techniques for servicing the elderly poor. For example, such a shift in attention has led to an appreciation of the client's social world and to the development of treatment strategies that engage their social linkages. Such approaches have taught therapists to comprehend clients' behavior in terms of their location within a social network system. The following case illustrates this type of network analysis.

Mr. C., a sixty-five-year-old man, periodically came to the Senior Outreach Program staff at the end of the month asking for loans so that he could purchase food and other necessities. Mr. C. admitted that his budgetary difficulties stemmed from his gambling at a local betting parlor. Initially, staff concentrated on Mr. C.'s problems with impulse control and his seemingly immature personality structure. However, when his social network was mapped, the staff discovered that Mr. C.'s entire social world revolved around the betting parlor. Moreover, many of his contacts frequently provided Mr. C. with loans, food, and other assistance. In delineating Mr. C.'s network, the team was able to reframe his behavior in terms of a social context that offered advantages as well as disadvantages, rather than in terms of psychopathology in Mr. C.

The use of network analysis requires a systems perspective. In other words, in network analysis, "symptoms, defenses, character structure, and personality are regarded as terms describing the individual's typical interaction which occurs in response to particular context, rather than as intrapsychic entities" (Jackson, 1967, p. 140). Network strategies, of course, should not be seen as replacing intrapsychic or dynamic models but rather as complementing them.

One network approach developed for use with older persons living in the community has involved strategic interventions with various components of the client's social matrix (Cohen and Sokolovsky, 1981). Such strategies include assisting network members to increase support and exchange within their existing system, helping clients to expand their networks, identifying and training natural neighborhood helpers (such as letter carriers or hotel maids) in how to assist the older person, and educating other service personnel in how to work with existing networks. A second approach has entailed the actual convening of all the key members of the elderly individual's social network—friends, relatives, service professionals—into a network "session" aimed at developing a treatment plan for the client, created and encouraged by the members themselves (Garrison and Howe, 1976).

Another focus beyond the arena of individual therapy has been to stimulate the growth of self-help or mutual-aid groups. Biegel, Shore, and Gordon (1984) identified three major types: formal self-help groups that meet for mutual support and guidance, formalized barter or service exchange programs, and programs that create artificial networks among the elderly to augment the exchange of assistance. Mutual-aid groups have been seen as a way to prod the elderly person out of her or his dependency role into a more proactive posture and to encourage him or her to ally with others in accomplishing goals. Moreover, because many groups are intergenerational, they help to break down age barriers and stereotypes.

Finally, advocacy groups go beyond the assistance of immediate support networks and mutual-aid groups to mobilize resources—political, economic, and attitudinal—to meet the needs of members (Biegel, 1984). An example of such a group is the Gray Panthers. This organization aims at making social change through social actions. Its goals include attacking ageism, creating coalitions with other groups for social and political change, and humanizing society. Similarly, the Community Service Society helped develop the Caregivers Network, a consumer advocacy group that has presented testimonies at public hearings, lobbied legislators, and sensitized professionals and the media to their unmet needs and burdens (Biegel, Shore, and Gordon, 1984). When therapists encourage their patients to take part in this kind of group activity, the effect can be quite therapeutic.

Conclusion

The earliest apostles of the community psychiatry movement recognized that all therapy must integrate the social context into individual treatment. Consequently, new therapies and techniques began to surface. Unfortunately, retrenchments in social programs over the past fifteen years deflected the focus of community psychiatry so that the "community" in community psychiatry has been largely submerged. Moreover, the elderly were not included in any significant way in the original community psychiatry movement. Hence, only the most rudimentary therapeutic techniques have been developed for those elderly served by public programs.

As public psychiatry programs for the elderly begin to emerge, we must refine our theories and techniques to serve this population better. We must create a broadened definition of psychotherapy that will incorporate work with social networks, mutual-aid groups, and advocacy groups. Similarly, clinicians must learn to recognize how social structures not only affect the daily activities but also penetrate the unconscious, the psychic defenses, and the cognitive styles of their patients. For many clinicians, such recognition may lead to a departure from more traditional methods. Kupers (1981), in a seminal work, suggested some of these ideas. Therapeutic endeavors with the elderly treated in public settings have the potential to alter radically the theoretical and clinical models that are typically employed with this age group. For this reason, clinicians working in public psychiatry serve not only as therapists but also as explorers.

References

Biegel, D. E. "Social Support Networks and the Care of the Elderly." In W. J. Sauer and R. T. Cloward (eds.), *Social Support Networks and the Care of the Elderly*. New York: Springer, 1984.

Biegel, D. E., Shore, B. K., and Gordon, E. *Building Support Networks for the Elderly*. Beverly Hills, Calif.: Sage, 1984.

Brown, E. R. "Medicare and Medicaid: The Process, Value, and Limits of Health Care Reforms." In M. Minkler and C. L. Estes (eds.), *Readings in the Political Economy of Aging*. Farmingdale, N.Y.: Baywood, 1984.

Butler, R. N. *Why Survive? Being Old in America*. New York: Harper & Row, 1975.

Butts, H. F., and Schachter, J. S. "Psychotherapy and Social Stratification: An Empirical Study of Practice in a Psychiatric Outpatient Clinic." *Journal of the American Psychoanalytic Association*, 1968, *16*, 792-808.

Cohen, C. I., and Sokolovsky, J. "Social Networks and the Elderly: Clinical Techniques." *International Journal of Family Therapy*, 1981, *3*, 281-294.

Estes, C. L., Swan, J. H., and Gerard, L. E. "Dominant and Competing Paradigms in Gerontology: Toward a Political Economy of Aging." In M. Minkler and C. L. Estes (eds.), *Readings in the Political Economy of Aging*. Farmingdale, N.Y.: Baywood, 1984.

Fanon, F. *Black Skin, White Masks*. New York: Grove Press, 1967.

Freire, P. *Education for Critical Consciousness*. New York: Continuum, 1987.

Freud, S. "On Psychotherapy." In J. Strachey (ed.), *The Complete Psychological Works of Sigmund Freud*. Vol. 7. London: Hogarth Press, 1957. (Originally published 1904.)

Garrison, J. E., and Howe, J. "Community Intervention with the Elderly: A Social Networks Approach." *Journal of the American Geriatrics Society*, 1976, *24*, 329-333.

Halleck, S. L. *The Politics of Therapy*. New York: Science House, 1971.

Jackson, D. D. "The Individual and the Larger Contexts." *Family Process*, 1967, *6*, 139-147.

Kane, R. L., Ouslander, J. G., and Abrass, I. B. *Essentials of Clinical Geriatrics*. New York: McGraw-Hill, 1984.

Kupers, T. A. *Public Therapy: The Practice of Psychotherapy in the Public Mental Health Clinic*. New York: Free Press, 1981.

Lazarus, L. W., and Sadavoy, J. "Psychotherapy with the Elderly." In L. W. Lazarus (ed.), *Essentials of Geriatric Psychiatry*. New York: Springer, 1988.

Minkler, M. "Blaming the Aged Victim: The Politics of Retrenchment in Times of Fiscal Conservatism." In M. Minkler and C. L. Estes (eds.), *Readings in the Political Economy of Aging*. Farmingdale, N.Y.: Baywood, 1984.

Myers, J. K., Weissman, M. M., Tischer, G. L., Holzer, C. E., Leaf, P. J., Orvaschel, H., Anthony, J. C., Burke, J. D., Kramer, M., and Stoltzman, R. "Six-Month Prevalence of Psychiatric Disorders in Three Communities." *Archives of General Psychiatry*, 1984, *41*, 959-967.

Navarro, V. "The Political Economy of Government Cuts for the Elderly." In M. Minkler and C. L. Estes (eds.), *Readings in the Political Economy of Aging*. Farmingdale, N.Y.: Baywood, 1984.

Rowe, J. W., and Kahn, R. L. "Human Aging: Usual and Successful." *Science*, 1987, *237*, 143-149.

Ryan, W. *Blaming the Victim*. New York: Vintage Books, 1971.

Sadavoy, J., and Leszcz, M. (eds.). *Treating the Elderly with Psychotherapy*. Madison, Wisc.: International Universities Press, 1987.

Salzman, C. *Clinical Geriatric Psychopharmacology*. New York: McGraw-Hill, 1984.

Talbott, J. A. "The Chronic Mentally Ill: What Do We Now Know and Why Aren't We Implementing What We Know?" In W. W. Menninger and G. T. Hannah (eds.), *The Chronic Mental Patient*. Vol. 2. Washington, D.C.: American Psychiatric Press, 1987.

Terestman, N., Miller, J. D., and Weber, J. J. "Blue-Collar Patients at a Psychoanalytic Clinic." *American Journal of Psychiatry*, 1974, *131*, 261-266.

U.S. General Accounting Office. *The Elderly Remain in Need of Mental Health Services*. Document no. HRD-82-112. Washington, D.C.: U.S. Government Printing Office, 1982.

Yesavage, J. A., and Karasu, T. B. "Psychotherapy with Elderly Patients." *American Journal of Psychiatry*, 1982, *36*, 41-55.

Carl I. Cohen is professor of psychiatry and director of geriatric psychiatry at the State University of New York Health Science Center, Brooklyn.

To be effective with working people, psychotherapeutic insights must be applied in a context that includes an understanding of work-related issues and their psychological impact on the individual.

Issues of Work, Workers, and Therapy

Lee Schore

Work and the conditions that surround it are a central and defining part of human life that shape and condition both daily activity and consciousness. The impact of work on workers' lives has not been given sufficient attention in traditional therapy, and as a result most workers have remained outside the "mental health" arena. The Center for Working Life (CWL), a nonprofit mental health agency that grew out of the work of the Institute for Labor and Mental Health (Lerner, 1986), develops training and education programs in collaboration with unions, organizes joint labor-management projects, and provides direct services that address the mental health needs of workers. In this chapter, I will discuss some reasons for the ineffectiveness of traditional psychotherapy with workers, outline some of the insights and theoretical formulations underlying the work of CWL, mention ways in which psychodynamic principles and the practice of therapy can be adapted to this kind of work, and provide an example of the application of the center's approach.

The Ineffectiveness of Traditional Therapy Models with Workers

Because traditional long-term intensive therapy does not take worker culture and the special needs of workers in a therapeutic setting into account, this model has been ineffective in helping workers. Historically, working-class men and women, particularly blue-collar workers, have underutilized mental health services, even when these services were fully covered in negotiated benefits.

One reason for this is the cultural stigma attached to using mental health services. In middle-class culture, going to a therapist may be seen as an opportunity for growth and increased self-knowledge, but in the working class it may be perceived as a sign of failure. Having to pay a stranger to listen to you talk about personal problems is considered "weird" and implies that you have no friends or family to rely on and that you can't handle things on your own.

When a worker does find his or her way into a therapist's office, it is usually at the insistence of some external authority, such as the courts, a doctor, or a work-mandated referral. Too often the interaction is unsatisfactory, and workers don't stay long. They report that they didn't understand their therapists or that the therapists didn't understand them. When a therapist does not consider work a valid subject for exploration and wants to move on to the "real issues," the client feels that his or her concerns and experience are being invalidated.

Workers usually come to therapy or "counseling" to deal with a specific problem. They may fear losing their job, or they may feel that their supervisor is driving them crazy. They may feel that they can't continue to work because of problems they are facing on the job, or they may seek help because one of their children is using drugs. In this context, traditional psychodynamic psychotherapy that emphasizes examination of the therapeutic relationship seems foreign.

For example, one woman seen at the Center for Working Life commented on her only other visit to a therapist, one that took place because she had been depressed since her husband's death. She entered the room. The therapist smiled and said nothing. She did not indicate where the client should sit or how to begin. The woman was uncomfortable and finally asked if she could sit down, waiting for the therapist to begin. After about ten minutes, the woman attempted to break the silence and ease her discomfort by looking around the room and finding something to say "to break the ice." She told me, "I didn't know if she was new at this and didn't know what to do or if she was just having a bad day. So, I tried to make it easier and told her I liked the picture she had on the wall. Well, she then went on to ask me a lot of questions about what I saw in the picture and finally told me that asking about the picture was my way of avoiding talking about myself. Can you beat that? Did she really think I came there to talk about her picture? She never even asked me anything about me. I was just being polite, just trying to start conversation. She was just rude; she didn't even try to welcome me into her place or make me feel comfortable there."

The Approach of the Center for Working Life

The Centrality of Work and Its Psychological Impact. At CWL we believe that work, as a source of satisfaction and meaning, plays an important role in the overall construct of the individual's psychological well-being. In traditional therapy models, even when the stress that results from the organization and conditions of work are recognized as a potential source of emotional problems, the impact of these conditions on the physical and psychological well-being of workers is minimized, and the psychosocial effects are viewed as the individual problems of working people and their families.

For example, despite increased recognition of the seriousness of occupational stress, traditional methods of addressing this problem tend to rely on behavior modification or cognitive psychology models that ignore the management styles and working conditions that play a significant part in creating the stress. The approach tends to confirm the worker's feeling that the symptoms are entirely due to his or her own inner flaw. If we are to address the mental health needs of workers, we must incorporate an understanding of work and its effects on the psychology of the individual into the mental health interventions of therapists and clinical social workers (Schore, 1987). Exclusive focus on the psychodynamic aspects of a client's low self-esteem fails to take into account the reality of the worker's life situation. In contrast, Sennett and Cobb (1972), Lerner (1986), and Schumacher (1979) discuss ways in which unfortunate aspects of the organization of work can have detrimental effects on the emotional well-being of workers.

Whenever possible, CWL, in addition to its services to individuals, supports workers in exploring the possibility that there might be collective solutions to some of their problems, solutions that might permit them to assert greater control over their work situations and their lives. For instance, they are encouraged to pursue channels that are open to them to express their dissatisfaction with particular conditions at work, whether these involve the grievance procedure, labor-management negotiations, or some other process. This is not to say that social action is prescribed as an alternative to psychotherapy or that there is little hope for improvement in the worker's symptomatology if social action is not possible. Rather, it is a way to demonstrate to the workers in concrete terms that their psychological problems are related both to their own idiosyncratic inner issues and to objective circumstances that exist independent of their personal foibles. The point is not to substitute social action for introspection and psychotherapy, but rather to counter the symptomatic worker's tendency to blame himself or herself entirely, with a concomitant reduction in self-esteem.

The Fallacy of Individual Solutions. Therapy that is based on white middle-class values can easily ignore the realities of workers' lives and, as a result, may mistake awareness of a threatening reality for paranoia and may misread appropriate expressions of anger. More important, the values and assumptions of middle-class therapists can implicitly invalidate the reality of a worker's life or the class values supporting it.

The nature of traditional therapy implies that there are individual solutions and options available to all members of the society. The individual solution for workers dealing with a "work-related problem" may be to leave their place of work and find other employment. However, since all workers cannot exercise this option, the implicit message is that it is up to the individual to adjust to the conditions of his or her work. This also implies that workers must take care of themselves as individuals in isolation from other workers who may be experiencing the same problems. Because of this, one of the effects of the concept of individual solutions is to leave workers divided and weakened.

Approaches based on this concept of individual solutions do not take into account the possibility that changes in the reality of the external situation may be necessary to resolve a problem. Instead, people are expected to make and accept choices that are not truly acceptable. For example, a single mother who works at night may be forced to choose a decent job that can support her and her children but that forces her to leave them home alone. For other workers, the choice may be between having a lousy job or no job. These workers have little or no control over the alternatives that society has made available. To look only at the individual's condition, reaction, and choices is to deny the social and economic reality in which they are embedded (Briar, 1988).

Because individuals do not have the power to bring about large-scale structural changes in their conditions, much of the power of workers is in collective action. This collective power may be exercised in changing work conditions, in winning comparable-worth settlements, or in redesigning the way work is performed. Whatever the specifics, the result is more power for both the individuals and the groups involved.

The recognition that the specific problems and related psychological issues of workers are intimately linked to their work conditions changes the context of the therapeutic encounter. To incorporate this larger reality, therapists must occasionally abandon the narrow limits of the practice of psychodynamic psychotherapy and move from behind the shield of neutrality to participate in changing the conditions that are damaging the clients they are seeking to serve.

Given this reality, CWL attempts to use the knowledge of psychodynamics combined with an understanding of the world of work to develop proactive early interventions, to prevent some of the "hidden injuries of class" (Sennett and Cobb, 1972), and to develop programs that will help workers understand the environment they are in and the effect that it has.

Adapting Psychotherapeutic Approaches

Having argued that traditional long-term psychotherapy is not a useful mode of intervention with a working-class population, I will also argue that to develop programs that are effective and accessible requires a clear understanding of the psychodynamic concerns that are being activated in each situation. Psychodynamic training is essential as a foundation for understanding human behavior and as a tool for distinguishing between a healthy response to a crisis and a pattern of pathology. In order for psychotherapy to meet the needs of working people, however, psychotherapeutic training must be expanded to include the following: socioeconomic, class, race, and gender issues that mold early childhood development; an approach to therapy based on an understanding of work conditions and class culture that validates the worker's experience; and new treatment strategies and modalities that make therapy more physically accessible and intellectually familiar.

The staff of the Center for Working Life is composed of licensed clinicians, interns, and educators who in addition to their professional training, all have some experience in blue- or white-collar jobs and involvement in labor unions. The integration of a knowledge of psychodynamics with the direct experience and understanding of the world of work is at the core of the center's approach. The center's services include union-based membership assistance programs (MAPs) and a social support model that combines counseling with job training and placement programs for workers who have lost their jobs due to plant closings or mass layoffs. This model is also used to introduce a counseling component into workplace literacy programs. The MAPs and the social support programs provide group experiences and make individual and family counseling sessions available. They also provide workshops on specific issues, such as stress, parenting, and substance abuse awareness. The experience gained in all these activities is then used to develop preventive mental health services for both employed and unemployed workers. The keys to providing these services include removing the stigma from them and making them accessible. This often means providing services in nontraditional ways and in nontraditional places, such as union halls, coffee shops, and people's homes. Thus, in working with workers, CWL finds that what is needed is a flexible and creative application of psychotherapeutic insights to the specific problems that arise in the context of workers' lives.

An Example: Dislocated Workers' Support Services

A worker becomes "dislocated" when he or she experiences job loss as a result of a plant closure or major downscaling. Dislocation is not the result of temporary economic cycles but reflects a permanent restructuring of the economy. Most dislocated workers cannot expect to return to a similar job with similar wages and benefits.

Because of this, the psychological impact of a plant closure goes far beyond the simple shock of losing a job. For many it is the end of a way of life and the loss of the "American dream." It creates a complex life crisis reaction that may involve an experience of loss, a time of mourning and grief, an identity crisis brought on by a sudden change of one's place in the world, a loss of self-esteem and a denial of self-worth, a profound rupture in trust, a sense of betrayal and abandonment, a shattering of a belief system, the disruption of an established family structure, a threat to family security, and an experience of real and righteous anger.

The process of adjustment to this new situation can be complex and difficult, stretching the economic and psychological resources of those affected. Some workers will not survive this experience without major life disruption, but given appropriate help in a timely fashion, the majority will.

As pointed out earlier, support and mental health services, to be effective, must be accessible, they must be part of the ordinary structure of the worker's experience, and they must be provided in a destigmatized way. All counseling contacts, from the most formal to the most casual, must be animated by a clear affirmation of the worth and dignity of the people involved. The anger that these people are experiencing, which is too often seen as a purely psychodynamic issue in traditional therapy, must be validated and given a safe and supportive environment for expression. Another critically important part of providing these services is the inclusion of a group experience, providing support and helping workers understand what they are feeling, why they are feeling it, and that they are not alone in feeling it. The group experience is essential in breaking down the worker's sense of isolation and self-blame (Schore, 1984).

To achieve these goals, CWL has participated in dislocated worker programs where counseling services are provided as an integral part of a job services and retraining program. CWL staff work side by side with job developers and job specialists and participate in such group functions as orientations, job-search workshops, and weekly ongoing job clubs.

The presence of clinical staff in all aspects of job services allows the psychodynamic intervention to be delivered in the context of other services that are being received by all workers in the program. To receive these services does not require that people identify themselves as needing help or that they go into a strange and, for them, stigmatized environment to receive it. Dealing with problems in this way moves the therapeutic encounter from a context of identified personal failure to one that allows the client to view the situation as an understandable reaction to a difficult situation. The role of the weekly job club is also critical in destigmatizing interventions. The job club is a group of eight to twenty-five workers who gather to talk about their job-hunting experiences and to get job leads. As cofacilitators, CWL staff help move the participants from internalized blame ("I am lazy, I am not employable, no one wants me, I have no value"), to a shared feeling of anger ("they used us and threw us away"), to a stronger sense of regaining control in their lives ("they controlled my life long enough, I'm not going to let them control it now, I'm going to get some training, and I'm going to get back what they took away all these years").

Counselors can intervene to reduce self-blame by helping workers understand that what they are experiencing is not so much a personal or individual failure to cope with a situation but an experience shared by everyone there. The workers' feelings and reactions are normalized by the therapist's reflections. For example, the therapist might say, "Having difficulty figuring out what to do now is not because you can't figure it out right but because you are not being given enough information to make important decisions," or "It's not that *you* are confused—we are *all* confused because it's truly confusing," or "A lot of families will go through hard times now—after all, the whole family has been laid off and their lives have also just been turned upside down by somebody else's decision."

These kinds of interventions restore dignity, remove self-blame, and leave workers feeling that they are understood, not blamed, and that it is safe to talk. A statement by the facilitator of what is being felt by most of the participants in the group usually leads to a group discussion that helps the participants recognize that they are not alone in what they are feeling and in the problems they are dealing with. After the job club meeting, many of the workers will initiate individual contact with the clinical staff. These contacts frequently turn into ongoing individual sessions focused on some particular aspect of the worker's difficulties.

Conclusion

Balancing an understanding of the psychological needs of clients with an understanding of their social and cultural context is essential to designing effective interventions. However, designing effective interventions is not enough. The insight and experience of therapists and mental health workers must also be used to design programs, shape public policy, and actively engage in the business of building a world consistent with our understanding of what is needed for the nurture and growth of productive human lives. Fanon (1967) pointed out many years ago that it is impossible to be truly healthy in an unhealthy society. The final test of our work is whether we contribute to the healing of our society as well as to the healing of our clients. In this larger context, working to ensure justice in our society is, in many ways, the best possible mental health intervention.

References

Briar, K. *Social Work and the Unemployed.* Silver Spring, Md.: National Association of Social Workers, 1988.

Fanon, F. *Black Skin, White Masks.* New York: Grove Press, 1967.

Lerner, M. P. *Surplus Powerlessness.* Oakland, Calif.: Institute for Labor and Mental Health, 1986.

Schore, L. "The Fremont Experience: A Counseling Program for Dislocated Workers." *International Journal of Mental Health,* 1984, *13* (12), 154–168.

Schore, L. "The Mental Health Effects of Work: An Issue for Social Work Education." *Catalyst,* 1987, *21,* 43–50.

Schumacher, E. F. *Good Work.* New York: Harper & Row, 1979.

Sennett, R., and Cobb, J. *The Hidden Injuries of Class.* New York: Random House, 1972.

Lee Schore is the executive director of the Center for Working Life in Oakland, California. She also serves as a consultant for various unions and dislocated worker programs.

As resources dwindle, mental health practitioners are forced to treat more difficult cases in a briefer time frame. A clinical strategy is presented for accomplishing some of this aim, and a note of caution is offered about going along happily with the trend.

Public Therapy in the Nineties: Too Tough Cases, Too Few Resources, Too Little Time

Terry A. Kupers

I recently conducted a training session on brief therapy for clinicians in the outpatient clinic of a county mental health department. I explained the selection criteria established by the pioneers of brief therapy and their recommendation that anyone who is severely disturbed, suicidal, has a history of substance abuse, or is unmotivated for therapy be excluded, since outcome studies demonstrate that brief therapy works poorly with these populations (Malan, 1976; Davanloo, 1978; Sifneos, 1972). The staff responded that they understand the clinical rationale for these selection criteria but that I should understand their department's mandate to limit the number of therapy sessions for adults to twelve, no matter what the degree of psychopathology. The most disturbed individuals in their caseloads might also be followed by case managers, but I must realize that the case managers are overworked, so in practice only the most severely disturbed patients with a long history of recidivism can be seen for more than twelve sessions. My task, then, was to teach the staff how to utilize a form of brief therapy that was designed for relatively functional and highly motivated clients with their caseloads of severely disturbed and relatively unmotivated ones.

Sadly, this scenario is neither accidental nor rare. These clinicians are not alone in having a mandate to treat tough cases in too little time. Whether it is a matter of dual diagnosis, of cases being referred from the criminal justice system, or merely of severe mental disorders, public mental health cases seem to be becoming more difficult. And with cutbacks in resources, time becomes the measure of fiscal accountability. Inpatient stays are reduced from months to weeks and then to days. Halfway houses and day-treatment programs that once worked with clients for a year or more are required to discharge them within six months or even three.

The problem is that for many of those who utilize public mental health programs, the trauma of parting or the dread of abandonment looms larger than any potential gain from psychotherapy. On the average, these clients are the least able to tolerate disappointments and partings of any kind and the most likely to experience graduation from a short-term program as abandonment. Consider the hospitalized patient who seems to do well on the inpatient unit, quickly responds to medications and milieu therapy, stops hallucinating and begins quickly to order his thoughts, is a work leader in ward meetings, becomes attached to his primary therapist, and seems motivated for independent living after discharge. As part of discharge planning, the primary therapist helps the patient make an appointment for a job interview. Suddenly, the night before the interview, the psychotic symptoms reappear and the patient becomes enraged at another patient, loses control, and the staff decide to lock him in a security room and raise the dosage of his neuroleptic medication.

Treatment tends to break down when the stay in a program ends, whether the program involves a stay in an inpatient unit, a residential setting, brief outpatient psychotherapy, or all of these in succession. When the time for termination arrives, many people with severe mental disorders fall apart in whatever way is typical for them. Some decompensate, some return to using drugs or alcohol, some stop complying with their regimen of prescribed medications, some become suicidal, and some merely experience an exacerbation of familiar symptoms. Consider a difficult client who is assigned to a psychology intern at a mental health clinic because no other staff have openings. The client, who has a history of multiple hospitalizations, begins to pull her life together. She moves from a transient hotel to an apartment, she reestablishes contact with her children who had been assigned to a foster home when their mother was last hospitalized, and she attends regular therapy sessions. After six months, the intern announces that the therapy will end in three months when the intern will be leaving the clinic. The woman says nothing. She politely says good-bye at the end of that session. The next day, she enters the clinic waiting room screaming obscenities, proceeds to tear up the room and throw the furniture around, and has to be readmitted to the hospital. We might dismiss this example as an unfortunate error in the selection of a case for an intern to see. But the time-limited design of community programs regularly confronts quite a few patients with the situation that is the most problematic for them: As soon as they feel connected with staff and familiar with the routine, it is time to leave. It is possible to recognize the pattern early, and there are ways to prevent some of its most destructive effects on treatment outcomes.

Before proceeding, I should comment on the way an unfortunate development is sometimes mistaken for a real opportunity. It is one thing for clinicians, confronted by an externally mandated time limit, to make the best of the situation by developing creative techniques to treat people in a briefer time frame, all the while protesting that it is inequitable and not the best way to conduct treatment. It is quite another to make an unfortunate restriction of services seem a virtue (Kupers, 1986). Too often clinicians are told that because of cutbacks in funding they will have to treat difficult clients in a shortened time frame, and they are asked to go along happily, even told that the innovations in therapeutic technique they come up with will be a boon to society; the advance press for brief therapy in public mental health clinics is a perfect example. Instead of clinicians "going along happily," I suggest a two-tiered approach: On the concrete clinical level, clinicians make the best of what resources there are and create new and better forms of treatment, but meanwhile, clinicians and consumers of mental health services join ranks in the public arena to demand more adequate funding for mental health services. I will begin with some thoughts about the clinical tier.

A Clinical Strategy

There are a group of chronically disabled individuals whose repeated decompensations, suicide attempts, or other symptoms of serious mental disorder tend to follow a pattern: Each decompensation or regression is preceded by what they perceive as a significant loss, rejection, separation, or betrayal. Often the pattern is not obvious, particularly if clinicians are not looking for it. For instance, a thirty-two-year-old man was arrested by the police for screaming loudly from his porch and threatening all passersby with physical violence. Discovering that the man was talking to himself and clearly hallucinating, the police brought him to the psychiatric emergency room. He was admitted and injected with neuroleptics. He had been an inpatient at the hospital on two prior occasions. There was a pattern: On each occasion, he had been in a stormy relationship with a wife or lover, she had threatened to leave, he had become abusive, she had left, and he had proceeded to drink, become full of rage, and decompensate. Of course, this pattern is often linked to a borderline character disorder (Kernberg, 1975; Masterson, 1976). Sometimes there is psychosis with coexisting borderline psychopathology (Gunderson and Elliott, 1985). But the pattern can also be detected in individuals assigned a diagnosis of severe mental disorder with no character pathology noted or in individuals in whom there is no major mental disorder. In any case, difficulty with partings is frequently part of the picture in the treatment of the seriously mentally ill.

Another patient in a state hospital was discharged six months after a serious suicide attempt. On her way out, in the lobby of the hospital, she proceeded to ingest all of the two weeks' medications she had been prescribed. Similarly, a certain number of residents in halfway houses seem to do well while in the house, and then when the time for termination nears, they regress and become symptomatic enough to require rehospitalization. Brief therapists in outpatient clinics often find that their patients do well during the beginning and middle phases of treatment; then their condition deteriorates as the date for termination nears.

In all of these settings, clinicians need to identify the people who are likely to present this kind of difficulty. I do a "history of partings." This includes not only looking at the obvious crises and decompensations that brought the client to the attention of the mental health system—the precipitating events for each admission to hospital or the events leading up to less serious "breakdowns"—but also a review of all significant partings over a lifetime. What was it like to leave home and enter daycare or kindergarten? What was it like to move to a new school? How was it for you when your parents divorced? When someone died? What was it like to graduate from one school and move on to the next, to break up with a girlfriend or boyfriend, to leave home, to lose a job, to end a marriage? A pattern is likely to emerge, a pattern that leads right up to the initial crisis or hospitalization and recurs through repeated contacts with the mental health system.

The next step is to point out this pattern and help the person see that it exists and that his or her particular way of coping with separations, losses, and disappointments is nonfunctional and self-destructive. Of course, this kind of insight is not always possible, and sometimes the clinician must use his or her wiles to help the person "get it." For instance, the patient who was just admitted to the hospital with a significant thought disorder is not likely to make such connections until he or she has calmed down or been stabilized on medications. The resident who is acting out and breaking rules in a halfway house is not likely to seek insight until some of the most self-destructive aspects of the rule breaking are confronted and he or she is feeling safe enough and trusting the staff enough to begin to wonder why the pattern is continually replayed. But whenever the individual is ready to begin understanding and to whatever extent, it is time to point out the pattern that is apparent in the history of partings and to suggest that there might be better ways to cope with the seemingly intolerable feelings and conflicts.

Next, it is time, early in the brief treatment, to point out that there is some potential for the pattern to recur even here (on the ward, in the day-treatment or halfway house program, in the supported employment program, in the clinic, and so on). In other words, the person will only be in this treatment for a limited amount of time, and then there will be another parting. How are we—the clinician (or the program) and the client—to work out a way to avoid a recurrence of the most unfortunate aspects of the pattern when the time arrives to end this segment of residence or treatment?

Ironically, it is one of the innovators in the type of brief therapy that specifically excludes the seriously mentally ill who provides this clue to working with the severely disturbed individual in a brief time frame. Mann's (1973; Mann and Goldman, 1982) twelve-session brief therapy is based on the assumption that most emotional symptomatology is related to the individual's difficulty in coping with separations, disappointments, and with the eventuality of death. In order to highlight this issue in the context of psychotherapy, he tells his patients in the first session that there are only eleven sessions remaining and asks how they feel about that. In the third session he reminds them that there are nine left, in the sixth that there are six, and so on. At each step, he explores the patient's reactions, including disappointment and other negative feelings about the therapist, and in the process forces the patient to confront and prepare for the fact that termination is coming. One can hope that the patient will work through enough of the issues related to termination to be able to benefit from the brief course of therapy.

Mann's strategy can be applied in treating the more seriously disturbed individual in psychotherapy, in the hospital, or in any of the community support modalities. I will present a schematic outline, but remember that there are idiosyncratic subtleties and complexities to its application in each case. First, be realistic and explicit about the limits of the treatment contract; maximizing the forewarning helps the patient avoid feeling seduced and abandoned. (Sometimes this kind of frankness merely gives the patient an opportunity not to bond so intensely with the staff—an opportunity he or she really ought to be afforded when there is a strict time limit.) Then, do a history of partings and point out the pattern that surfaces. Next, point out that in this treatment context, we have an opportunity to rework the pattern, since we will be parting at the end of the contracted time. Then, help the patient face the fact that we cannot accomplish everything, and some stones will be left unturned, while repeatedly reminding him or her that there are alternative approaches to coping with the feelings that result. Finally, try to help the client find ways to generalize the lessons of this treatment to experiences in other living situations, programs, and relationships that must eventually end.

I arrived at this general strategy while attempting to advise clinicians in an outpatient setting on the conduct of brief therapy with difficult patients. Effective utilization of the strategy can help the patient deal with a troubling and widespread aspect of his or her life-style: Because hospital and community support programs tend to be constructed in sequential segments, the patient's course in the mental health system tends to be punctuated by multiple terminations and entries into new situations. If he or she can learn from a brief therapy or time-limited program some slightly less destructive way to cope with loss or change, there is reason to hope that he or she will do better in other settings. Additionally, because chronic consumers of public mental health services tend to have difficulty establishing and maintaining long-term intimate relationships, they must learn to tolerate the rejections, betrayals, and losses that tend to be their plight. Further, being at the lowest rung of the socioeconomic ladder, their living situations tend to be transient and their financial security tenuous. In other words, chronic patients, who tend not to tolerate change well, find themselves having to cope with almost continual changes, including movement from one community support program to another or back to the hospital, the loss of intimates from relationships that seem to go repeatedly awry, and the loss of material comforts every time there is more financial hardship. Therapy and therapeutic programs that make use of the strategy I outlined can serve to prepare these clients for the repeated losses and traumas that go with the territory.

Implications for Program Design

The issues patients have about partings should be taken into account in the designing of mental health programs. Case management (Harris and Bergman, 1987) and the continuous-treatment team (Knoedler, 1989) are examples of innovations in design that, while probably not explicitly established with this strategy in mind, do serve to fill some of the gaps in mental health systems for the population I have been describing. These innovations permit a clinician, case manager, or psychiatrist to get to know and work with a patient over a long period of time. Alternatively, if the providers are able to offer the patient some sort of replacement for the lost provider or program and if some kind of transition can be arranged, the loss of the old relationship or situation and the beginning of the new are made that much easier. An example is the outpatient clinic where a trainee is scheduled to leave the clinic at a certain time, but because the treatment team feels that this would not be a good time for a particular patient to terminate psychotherapy, another trainee is asked to accept transfer of the case (Pumpian-Mindlin, 1958). Where possible, it helps to introduce the patient to the new therapist before the old one leaves. Where severe staff shortage is the reason for the limit to the length of therapy, this option might not be available. In either case, the strategy I have outlined can be usefully applied.

A recent consultation I conducted with the staff of a transitional apartment program is an example of a way to utilize the strategy I have outlined to fill gaps in community support programs. The staff complain that quite a few of the clients who are referred from halfway houses decompensate soon after arriving at the apartments. Of course, at the halfway house the clients are "spoon-fed." If they do not get up in the morning in time to go to day treatment or if they do not seem able to comply with their medications, the staff at the halfway house wake them or monitor their medications. At the transitional apartments, they are living with one or more roommates, and they only see a staff member once a week in an individual meeting and once at the weekly apartment group meeting.

The staff feel the clients are often ill prepared to leave the house they have been in for months, and there is an intolerable drop-off in the level of caretaking when they move to the apartments. The staff agree that their residents' problems fit the pattern I have presented here and that it would be helpful to figure out a way to apply the general strategy I have outlined. Together we find a way: For all residents of halfway houses in the vicinity who wish to move eventually to the transitional apartments, attendance will be required at two or three weekly orientation sessions on apartment living. The sessions will be conducted jointly by one staff member of the transitional apartments and one halfway house staff member. At the ongoing weekly preadmission orientation meetings, there will be a discussion about apartment living, education about the need to comply with medications, some tips on getting along with roommates, and so on. In effect, by attending the meetings, the resident will be given at least two or three weeks' notice about the impending move out of the halfway house, an education about apartment living, and an opportunity to work on the issues of parting and transition to a new setting. He or she might even meet someone at orientation who will be moving to the apartments at the same time. The staff of the apartments will have an opportunity to assess potential residents' coping skills and motivation to be in the apartments. And the staffs of all the programs will have an opportunity to collaborate and to learn about each others' work. This is just one example of the way in which psychodynamic principles can inform the design and structure of programs.

Of course, the halfway-house-to-transitional-apartments system I have been discussing is one in which the patient is made to traverse a sequence of time-limited programs on the road to independent living. The sad truth is that many patients never make it to this goal, always seeming to decompensate just when their providers are beginning to think they are ready for a new level of independence. The idea of weekly orientation meetings is merely a transitional strategy, a strategy for making a sequential system of community support programs more tolerable.

If a significant proportion of the seriously mentally ill fit the pattern I have been describing, then it is time to be more realistic, to stop designing programs with strict time limits that are aimed at graduation to independent living. Better than intensive short-term programs (hospital, day treatment, halfway house, and transitional apartments) would be longer-term, less intensive programs where the sole criterion of a successful treatment is not completion of the whole sequence. We are realizing that for many who have been deinstitutionalized or who came into the system after the closing of the large public psychiatric hospitals, independent living is probably an unrealizable goal. Better that these individuals should be supplied with a less staff-intensive mental health program but one that can continue to satisfy minimal needs indefinitely. In the Northeast, the supported housing programs that are being set up reflect some sensitivity to this issue (Blanch, Carling, and Ridgway, 1988). The resident stays put in a partially subsidized apartment or in the family home, while the number of mental health staff involved in supporting the patient rises and falls over time, depending on the patient's needs. Here I am supplementing the strategy I have outlined with the proviso that it would be better to design service delivery systems that make the strategy unnecessary. In other words, if we must work within strict time limits with clients who have difficulty tolerating changes and partings, then the strategy I outlined might prove invaluable. But it would be much better in many cases to redesign systems so that there are fewer time limits.

One of the problems I encounter when I teach brief therapy in public mental health clinics is that staff think they are a failure because they cannot achieve the happy outcomes the clinicians who write the books on brief therapy seem to achieve. It helps when I explain that they should not expect comparable results; their patients are much more severely disturbed and would be rejected as candidates for brief therapy in the clinics of most of the innovators. If public therapists are not reminded of this fact, they may experience burnout (Mendel, 1979; Kupers, 1981). Again, it is important to realize that some of the seriously mentally ill will never move on to truly independent living (Bachrach and Lamb, 1989). Some of them will continue to recycle in and out of hospitals (Solomon and Doll, 1979). Perhaps the goal for these people should not be independent living but rather a relatively stable and satisfying life in the community utilizing a minimum but adequate level of mental health resources over a long period of time.

The Public Arena

When budget cuts occur and there are less resources to accomplish difficult tasks, there are innovations. Providers are creative in designing new programs and approaches so that the populations they are assigned to serve will continue to be served well. The commitment, enthusiasm, and creativity of the innovators is inspiring. But too often an unfortunate cycle develops: Innovators devise ways to serve their clientele with fewer resources, and their funding agencies see that they are able to do more with less. Then, in the next round of budget decisions, the funding is diminished even further, the rationale being that the providers of services have done such a good job that it is clear they do not need a larger budget. The advent of brief therapy is a good example. Brief therapy was originally designed to permit therapists in busy clinics to skim the most treatable cases from their waiting lists, treat them quickly and efficiently, and thereby quickly reduce the number of people waiting for longer-term psychotherapy (Gustafson, 1986). But soon health plans, public administrations, and third-party payers began to mandate a limited number of sessions for all, using the rationale that there now existed a treatment modality that could accomplish as much as longer-term therapy but in significantly less time (Kupers, 1988).

Another example of this unfortunate cycle occurred in a county where a well-organized community group recently advocated setting up a residential program for the psychiatrically disabled of the inner city. The county would subsidize rents, but there would be little if any expense for staff since the community group would supply volunteers to staff the program. The program was a success in its first year. Then the county, in its next year's budget proposal, reduced the already thin mental health budget even further, claiming that by enlarging the successful community residential program the mental health system could reduce the number of staff needed to supply support services to the seriously mentally ill. In effect, the innovators—hardworking mental health staff and consumers— were being punished for their success.

I (Kupers, 1981) have pointed out some similarities between the public therapist's burnout and the chronic mental patient's inability to feel he or she will ever accomplish anything of merit. Both feel powerless to effect change in their circumstances. The chronic patient feels impotent and becomes lethargic. The underpaid practitioner feels a failure as a clinician or healer. Both blame themselves for their failures. I still believe: "It is only because of insecurity about their adequacy as therapists that very many more public therapists do not loudly protest the constraints the mental health system places on their ability to practice therapy" (p. 225).

One can hope that in the nineties more practitioners will realize that clinical failure is made more likely by budget cuts, and there will be less self-blame and burnout (Kupers, 1990). Dumont (1989) insists the public therapist must be an activist, the aim of Dumont's activism in recent years being to end lead poisoning in low-income communities. There is need for many forms of activism. For instance, mental health practitioners are beginning to ally with consumers and speak out publicly. While the American Psychiatric Association was holding its annual meeting in San Francisco May 8–12, 1989, there was a large demonstration in Sacramento. Busloads of mental patients, practitioners, and supporters converged on the state capitol for a day of protest. They demonstrated and lobbied for the restoration of mental health funds that the governor had cut from the state budget. Some A.P.A. members took a day off from the annual meeting to participate in the demonstration.

I have suggested a two-tiered response to the mandate to shorten treatment in many public mental health settings. In regard to the first tier, I have presented a clinical strategy. In regard to the second, the social dimension, it is clear that clinicians and consumers will have to join ranks and demand more adequate funding for mental health programs if quality mental health servicers are to be provided. This is the reality of the nineties.

References

Bachrach, L. L., and Lamb, H. R. "What Have We Learned from Deinstitutionalization?" *Psychiatric Annals*, 1989, *19* (1), 12–21.

Blanch, A. K., Carling, P. J., and Ridgway, P. "Normal Housing with Specialized Supports: Psychiatric Rehabilitation Approach to Living in the Community." *Rehabilitation Psychology*, 1988, *33* (1), 47–55.

Davanloo, H. (ed.) *Basic Principles and Techniques in Short-Term Dynamic Psychotherapy*. New York: Spectrum, 1978.

Dumont, M. P. "An Unfolding Memoir of Community Mental Health." *Readings*, Sept. 1989, pp. 4–7.

Gunderson, J. G., and Elliott, G. R. "The Interface Between Borderline Personality Disorder and Affective Disorder." *American Journal of Psychiatry*, 1985, *142*, 277–288.

Gustafson, J. P. *The Complex Secret of Brief Psychotherapy*. New York: Norton, 1986.

Harris, M., and Bergman, H. C. "Case Management with the Chronically Mentally Ill: A Clinical Perspective." *American Journal of Orthopsychiatry*, 1987, *57* (2), 296–302.

Kernberg, O. F. *Borderline Conditions and Pathological Narcissism*. New York: Aronson, 1975.

Knoedler, W. "The Continuous-Treatment Team Model: Role of the Psychiatrist." *Psychiatric Annals*, 1989, *19* (1), 35–40.

Kupers, T. A. "Staff Burnout." In T. A. Kupers, *Public Therapy: The Practice of Psychotherapy in the Public Mental Health Clinic*. New York: Free Press, 1981.

Kupers, T. A. "The Dual Potential of Brief Psychotherapy." *Free Associations*, 1986, *6*, 80–99.

Kupers, T. A. *Ending Therapy: The Meaning of Termination*. New York: New York University Press, 1988.

Kupers, T. A. "Big Ideas, and Little Ones." *Community Mental Health Journal*, 1990, *26* (3), 217–220.

Malan, D. H. *The Frontier of Brief Psychotherapy*. New York: Plenum, 1976.

Mann, J. *Time-Limited Psychotherapy.* Cambridge, Mass.: Harvard University Press, 1973.

Mann, J., and Goldman, P. *A Casebook in Time-Limited Psychotherapy.* New York: McGraw-Hill, 1982.

Masterson, J. F. *Psychotherapy of the Borderline Adult.* New York: Brunner/Mazel, 1976.

Pumpian-Mindlin, E. "Comments on Technique of Termination and Transfer in a Clinic Setting." *American Journal of Psychotherapy,* 1958, *12,* 455–564.

Sifneos, P. E. *Short-Term Dynamic Psychotherapy.* New York: Plenum, 1972.

Solomon, P., and Doll, W. "The Varieties of Readmission: The Case Against the Use of Recidivism Rates as a Measure of Program Effectiveness." *American Journal of Orthopsychiatry,* 1979, *4,* 230–239.

Terry A. Kupers practices psychiatry in Oakland, California, is on the faculty of The Wright Institute in Berkeley, and is a consultant to several community mental health agencies.

Index

Ordering Information

New Directions for Mental Health Services is a series of paperback books that presents timely and readable volumes on subjects of concern to clinicians, administrators, and others involved in the care of the mentally disabled. Each volume is devoted to one topic and includes a broad range of authoritative articles written by noted specialists in the field. Books in the series are published quarterly in Fall, Winter, Spring and Summer and are available for purchase by subscription as well as by single copy.

Subscriptions for 1990 cost $48.00 for individuals (a savings of 20 percent over single-copy prices) and $64.00 for institutions, agencies, and libraries. Please do not send institutional checks for personal subscriptions. Standing orders are accepted.

Single copies cost $14.95 when payment accompanies order. (California, New Jersey, New York, and Washington, D.C., residents please include appropriate sales tax.) Billed orders will be charged postage and handling.

Discounts for quantity orders are available. Please write to the address below for information.

All orders must include either the name of an individual or an official purchase order number. Please submit your order as follows:

 Subscriptions: specify series and year subscription is to begin
 Single copies: include individual title code (such as MHS1)

Mail all orders to:
 Jossey-Bass Inc., Publishers
 350 Sansome Street
 San Francisco, California 94104